Book Title: Light Sensitivity Pain Reduction Techniques For Electronic Devices

My pseudonym "Thecyclecasenumber Goalinventionsystemauthor" is in reference to a method of inventing goals which I created in a drawing journal in 2013. I wrote my first book from 2019-2021 entitled "*Goal Invention: The Mental Therapy, Sport, and Hobby*" which instructs "The Cycle Case Number Goal Invention System", the system that I enjoyed using from 2013 onwards.

Contact me at my emails:

goalinventionthebookfeedback@gmail.com

letssavecinemaproductions@gmail.com

I do not use any social media accounts other than a YouTube channel entitled, "Let's Save Cinema Productions".

Disclaimer: I am not a doctor, and this book is not medical advice. Seek consultation with a medical professional before applying any of the techniques featured in this book. Feel free to bring this book to your medical professionals/eye doctors to show them the techniques addressed in this book and ask them if the techniques in this book are right for you.
I am not legally responsible for the outcomes of readers if they choose to perform the techniques that are taught in this book.

Light Sensitivity Pain Reduction Techniques for Electronic Devices

By: Russel Alden Arlotta
Illustrated By Amungwa Linus 'Kayaman'
Cover Device Logos Created By Caitlin

Other Books Written By:
Russel Alden Arlotta & Illustrated By Amungwa Linus 'Kayaman'

- ***Goal Invention: The Mental Therapy, Sport, and Hobby (235 pages)***
- ***How Cellphones Cropped, Distorted, and Visually Censored Cinema: Let's Save Cinema (164 pages)***
- ***The Detective Show Directory (24 pages)***
- ***The U.K. Comedy Show Directory (30 pages)***

All Books Available on Amazon in Paperback and Digitally on Play Store's Book Section.

About The Author: Russel Alden Arlotta

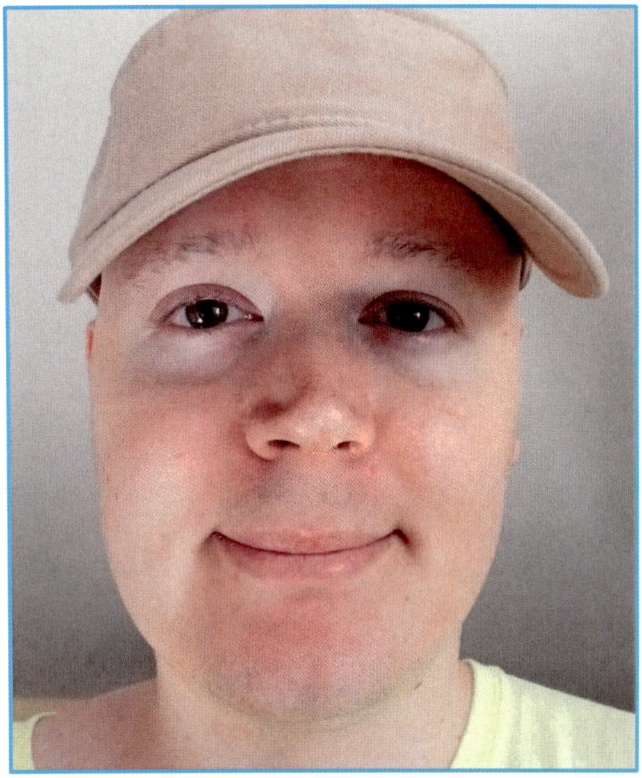

(A.K.A Thecyclecasenumber Goalinventionsystemauthor)

I graduated from Montgomery College. My most influential courses that I took from college, were *Introduction to College Writing* by Professor Matthew Decker, and *Introduction to Computer Applications* by Professor Joel Levine. Those courses alone provided me with the tools and skills to write all five of the books that I eventually would go on to write.
In 2013, I created a method of formulating goals in a drawing journal. I entitled the drawing journal's creation as *The Cycle Case Number Goal Invention System*. In 2019, I began writing my first book, "*Goal Invention: The Mental Therapy, Sport, and Hobby*", which instructs *The Cycle Case Number Goal Invention System* (and this is where my pseudonym originates).

Mr. Rolf Barber of Montgomery College has constantly supported me throughout my academia and my post academic writing career. Much of my academic studies were completed in the student research facility that was managed by Mr. Owen Powers of Montgomery College.
Mr. Wendi and Mr. Darrell supported me throughout my time at Montgomery College.
There are too many professors and staff to acknowledge who supported me throughout my academic career at MC, so I thank all the professors and staff that I have not mentioned by name.
Coach Kraig Kinsey supported me throughout my academic and writing career.
I thank Louie Tee of Louie Tee Network for his constant support and sports commentary.
Lastly, the vast majority of credit behind all my books and schooling is my parents, Joan and Russ, and my sisters, Allison, and Caitlin. With my family, my books are possible.
My extended family throughout my entire life has supported me unconditionally, thanks.

I dedicate this book to my mom, Joan Goodhue, and my dad, Russ Arlotta.

Me and my dad celebrating the finished product of this book in the summer of 2024.

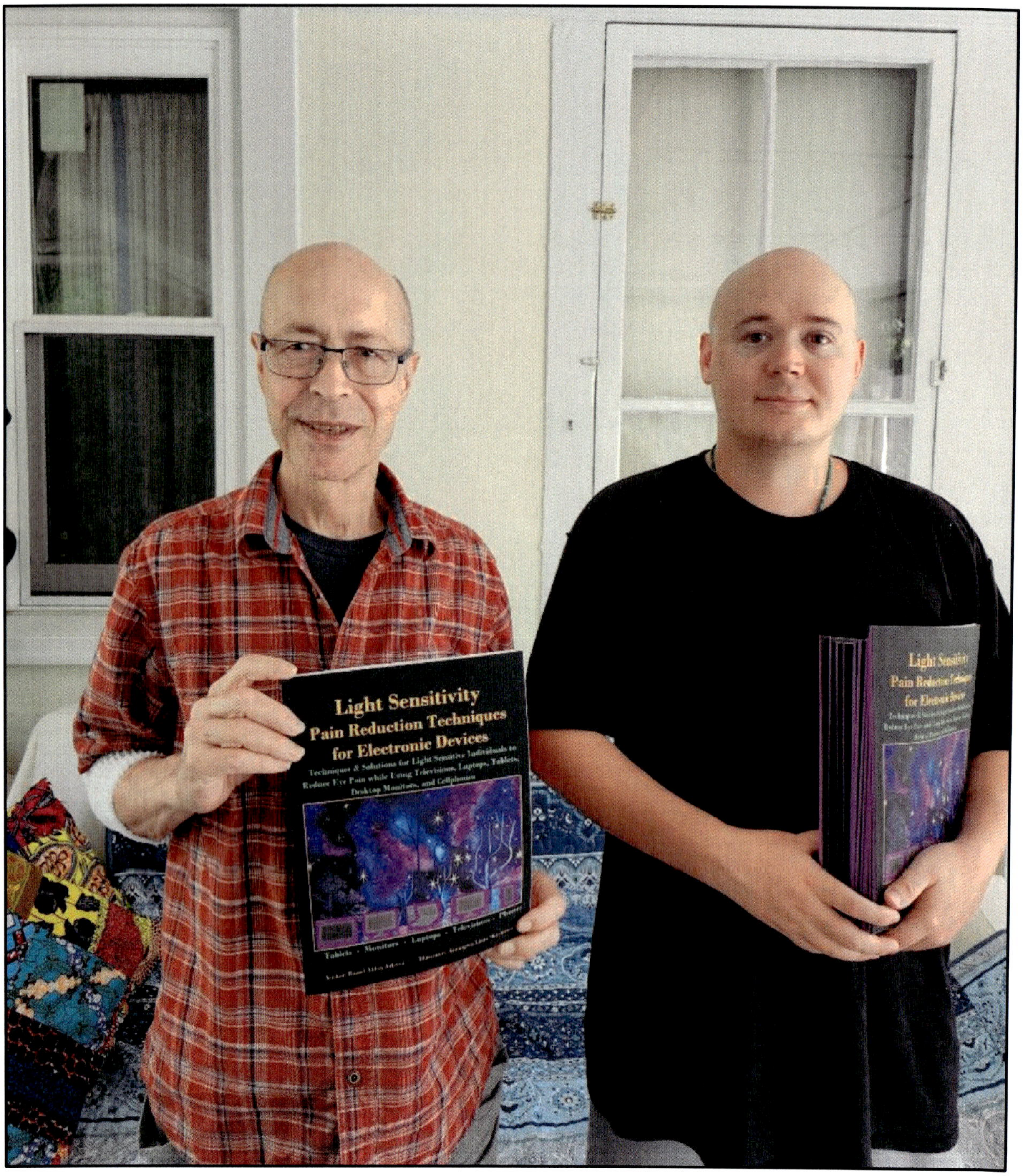

Author: Russel Alden Arlotta

Founder and Creator of the Goal Setting Workbook,

'The Cycle Case Number Goal Invention System' Est. 2013

And

Illustrator: Amungwa Linus 'KAYAMAN'

Presents

Light Sensitivity Pain Reduction Techniques For Electronic Devices

Let's Save Cinema Productions

Legal Disclaimer: *Light sensitivity conditions present many risks and challenges and requires care and collaboration with medical professionals and eye doctors.*
This book is not medical advice. I am not legally responsible for the outcomes of readers if they choose to perform the techniques that are taught in this book.
Please feel free to show this book to medical professionals and eye doctors and ask them if any of the techniques addressed in this book are right for you.

This book instructs techniques which helped me to reduce eye pains and discomfort from the usage of electronic devices due to a general light sensitivity condition caused from a sudden accident. The techniques featured in this book do not eliminate all eye pain & eye discomforts from light sensitivity conditions. Yet, I believe that the techniques addressed in this book can reduce the amount of eye pain & eye discomforts for most light sensitivity conditions.

One of the greatest barriers for individuals with chronic light sensitivity conditions in the modern world is the usage of electronics and artificial lights. This book focuses primarily on techniques to reduce eye pain and discomforts while using electronic devices such as televisions, laptops, cellphones, tablets, and monitors. While techniques can reduce the amount of pain and eye discomforts from light sensitivity conditions, some activities are especially difficult and cause too much eye pain to continue even with the usage of techniques.

In Chapter 1, I will begin this book by teaching the devices and activities that I had to quit completely in order to prevent significant eye pain and eye strain (of which some eye strains took weeks and months to recover from the eye pain). Following Chapter 1, I will instruct the individual techniques that I learned to reduce eye pain and eye discomforts while using each type of electronic device.
I would also like to note that with light sensitivity conditions, there are always limitations, sacrifices, and selective usages that must be applied to reduce the amount of eye pain and eye strains that may occur while using electronic devices.

Table of Contents

At the end of Chapter 2-5, I also include a blank template for the individual reader to create & document their own techniques and solutions for each electronic device.

This is because light sensitivity conditions vary, and individualized customized techniques may be needed.

I hope you enjoy reading this book, RAA

Chapter 1:

Disclaimer & Devices I Was Forced to Quit: Handheld Gaming Devices

Painter: Amungwa Linus 'Kayaman'

Chapter 1: Disclaimer & Devices I Was Forced to Quit: Handheld Gaming Devices

Disclaimer: I am not a doctor, and this is not medical advice. Seek consultation with a medical professional before applying any of the techniques featured in this book. Feel free to bring this book to your medical professionals and eye doctors to show them the techniques addressed in this book and ask them if the techniques in this book are right for you. I am not legally responsible for the outcomes of readers if they choose to perform the techniques taught in this book.

Disclaimer & Devices I was Forced to Quit: Handheld Gaming Devices.

Unfortunately, even with all the solutions addressed in this book, I was forced to quit handheld gaming, as the eye pain was too strong. With only 30 minutes of playing a handheld gaming device, a strong eye strain occurred with both eyes. It took 2 months for the eye pain to heal and subside. Even worse, from that incident my eyes became even more susceptible to light sensitivity. One of the real risks and dangers of chronic light sensitivity conditions is that chronic inner eye pain and strains can occur and cause eye pain which takes weeks and months for the eye pain to subside. I start this book with Chapter 1 to state that the techniques in this book reduce eye pain for some activities (but not all) and that compromises are a part of the process of dealing with light sensitivity conditions.

For handheld gaming, my compromise was hooking up handheld gaming devices to TVs and monitors (see the TV and monitor section of Chapter 4), as it is much easier on the eyes to look at screens from far away. Furthermore, I quit most videogames and played primarily only one game that I could easily play without plot called skater xl (story games are difficult to play with chronic light sensitivity conditions), as the solutions to reduce eye pain make it difficult to see text and some of the objects and scenes on the screen of a videogame.

Chronic light sensitivity conditions cause constant fear of setbacks and unfortunately setbacks are a difficult reality that must be approached with great care. Eye strains and eye pains can occur from light sensitivity conditions in which the eye pains last days, weeks, or even months until the eye pain subsides.

Chapter 1: Disclaimer & Devices I Was Forced to Quit: Handheld Gaming Devices Continued…

I start this book off with the difficult reality that there are no cures for most chronic light sensitivity conditions. Anything that causes eye pain should be stopped immediately and further modified with custom techniques so that the activity does not cause eye pain.

Individuals with light sensitivity conditions should take great care and work with medical professionals before attempting any of the techniques addressed in this book.

Please feel free to show this book to medical professionals and especially to eye doctors and ask them if the techniques addressed in this book are right for you.

Fortunately, many activities that cause eye pain for individuals with light sensitivity conditions can be greatly reduced with customized techniques and solutions. For the last few years, I tried all that I could to work around a general chronic light sensitivity condition. Through this small book, I hope to provide additional help to individuals with chronic light sensitivity conditions.

End of Chapter 1.

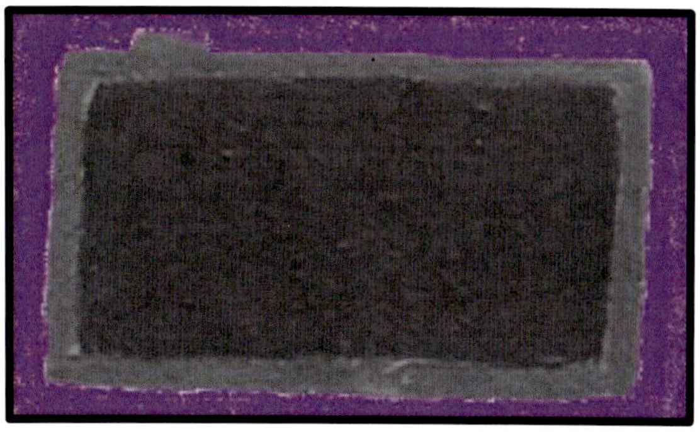

Chapter 2:
Tablets

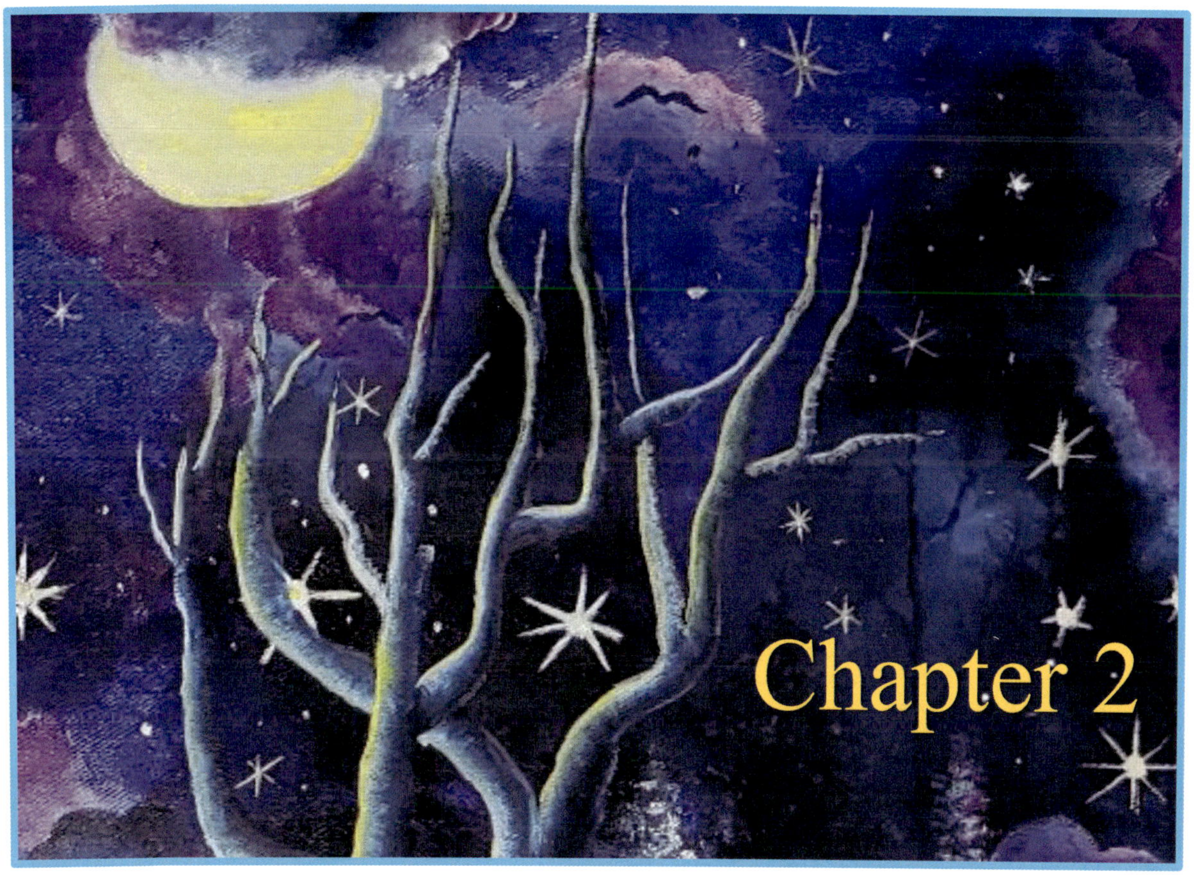

Painter: Amungwa Linus 'Kayaman'

Chapter 2 Tablets:

I am beginning Chapter 2, by previewing the format of Chapter 2 and also Chapters 3, 4, and 5.

By previewing the format of this chapter and the other remaining chapters, I believe that this book will be of greater use to the reader.

In Chapter 2 – Chapter 5, I present in detail the process of finding a solution to reduce eye pain while using each respective electronic device.

In Chapter 2 – Chapter 5, I also present the solution I developed and then I present that same solution in combination with another solution that I later discovered. I credit both solutions discussed in this book in combination with one another as being the primary solutions which enabled me to reduce eye pain while using tablets and other electronic devices.

I will now present for Chapter 2, the solutions that I developed and discovered to reduce eye pain while using tablets.

Chapter 2 Tablets

Origins: Several years ago, a sudden small accident caused a chronic light sensitivity condition. From that situation, I had to quit tablets and all electronic devices for about 3 months until I created techniques to enable me to use tablets and electronic devices.

Solution: It took about 3 months to find a solution. During that time, I wrote by hand (on a notebook) the draft of my second book *"How Cellphones Cropped, Distorted, and Visually Censored Cinema: Let's Save Cinema"*. During those 3 months of trial and error, I bought and tried dozens of sunglasses (anti blue light & regular sunglasses etc.). Unfortunately, all the sunglasses that I tried did not reduce eye pain while using tablets. Following that attempt, I tried various anti blue light screens placed on my tablet. Yet again, the anti-blue light screens placed on the tablet did not reduce the amount of eye pain while using the tablet.

After several months of failed attempts to reduce eye pain while using tablets, I thought of a solution which involved stacked privacy screens placed over the tablet with kinesiology tape. I bought multiple privacy screens and custom fit them to the size of my tablet. I then used a wireless (or wired) mouse for my tablet as the tablet's touch screen does not work with stacked privacy screens. Fortunately, my idea was correct and after adding 6 privacy screens stacked on the tablet, I was able to significantly reduce the amount of eye pain and discomfort that occurs while using tablets. Four months after the sudden accident, I was able to watch shows and movies on my tablet again (albeit with limited visibility due to the darkening effect of privacy screens). While the pain was significantly reduced, it took me one year to implement natural light to reduce the eye pain even more.

Solution + Natural Light: I was so excited to be able to watch shows and movies again. Even though the visibility is not great with the stacked privacy screens on the tablet's screen, I can make out the majority of the scenes of shows and movies on the tablet. While the solution reduced the eye pain, I was still dealing with mild to moderate eye pains while using tablets. The solution reduced eye pain significantly while using tablets, but it would take another year for me to discover the usage of daytime's natural light to reduce eye pain even more while using tablets. A year after the accident, I made the decision to experiment with natural light by using my tablet with the 6 stacked privacy screens near my window's natural light. This experiment proved successful and it reduced the amount of eye pains that occurred while using tablets.

Chapter 2 Tablets Continued...

Solution + Natural Light Continued: By adding the tablet on a table near a window in the daytime and watching my tablet with 6 stacked privacy screens, I was able to reduce the amount of eye pains and eye strains that occurred while using tablets. For these reasons, I primarily use tablets and all electronics in the day near a window and I stop using electronics in the evening and nighttime. The natural light of daytime in combination with 6 stacked privacy screens reduced the amount of eye pain and eye strains that occurred while using tablets.

The only issue that occurred was the varying amounts of natural light. On cloudy days, the amount of natural light was fine and stable, and I could see the tablet clearly. However, at some points in time during sunny days, I could not see the screen very well. For sunny days, I thought of using a wall divider with a simple bed sheet to place on the wall divider in front of the window. With the usage and adjustments of the wall divider (with an ambient colored bed sheet placed over the wall divider), I could customize the amount of natural light needed each day. A foam board can be used instead of a wall divider.

It is important to note however that on sunny days, I do not use wall dividers or foam boards on sunny days all the time. For example, on sunny days, I mostly use my tablet near a window without using a wall divider/foam board. Depending on where the sun is and where your windows are, you may not need to use a wall divider/foamboard.

On sunny days, I particularly only use the wall divider/foamboard in the afternoon when the sun is facing directly at my windows (in order to control the amount of natural light). The goal is to get as much possible natural light while still being able to see the contents of the screen on the tablet. On sunny days, I enjoy using my tablet lying down near a window without a wall divider/foamboard for most of the day. On cloudy days, I enjoy using the tablet while lying down near a window (without a wall divider/foamboard) throughout the entire day because cloudy days provide constant and mild natural light. Again, a wall divider/foamboard may only be needed when the sun is facing directly at the window, which could only be within a few hours' time frame.

It is also important to note that I used an amazon basics mouse (wireless or wired) and an amazon basics wireless USB to tablet converter, so that the wireless/wired mouse would work (the wireless Amazon Basics USB to tablet converter works for both a wired and wireless mouse).

Chapter 2 Tablets Continued...

It is also important to note that stacked privacy screens sometimes create waves of lines. This can be solved for most privacy screens by switching the side of the privacy screen to the other side so that no squiggly lines or waves appear. It will take a little bit of time to figure out the placement of privacy screens so that the privacy screens don't cause lines and waves. I personally used a variety of privacy screens, and then used a combination that did not cause waves and lines by switching the privacy screens' sides until no squiggly lines/waves appeared.

Before I present the instructions on how to install privacy screens to a tablet, I would like to first clarify and explain exactly what a privacy screen is.

Clarification of a Privacy Screen:

It is important to note the difference of a privacy screen and an anti-blue light screen. Anti-blue light screens were intended to filter out blue light from screens once placed on electronic devices. For me, anti-blue light screens did not reduce my eye pain for any device.

The clear ineffective ability for anti-blue light screens to reduce eye pain for many individuals with chronic light sensitivity conditions compelled me to create this clarification section of the difference between "privacy screens" and "anti-blue light screens".

Privacy screens were invented and intended to be used for workers and individuals at the workplace or at coffee stores to be able to put a privacy screen on their devices, so that nearby people would not be able to see the contents of their screens from the left or right side of the devices. Privacy screens work by only being able to see the contents of the screen if one is looking directly straight on at a screen with a privacy screen placed on it.

Privacy screens were not intended to reduce eye pain for individuals with light sensitivity conditions; however, when multiple privacy screens are stacked together and placed on a screen, the privacy screens generally do make the usage of electronics less painful to the eyes for light sensitive individuals. The unintended pain reducing effect of placing multiple stacked privacy screens on devices' screens is vital information for individuals with chronic light sensitivity conditions.

Step 1 Tablets: Custom fit your privacy screens to the desired size of your tablet's screen size and pick your desired amount of privacy screens stacked on each other (from 2-6) depending on preference. For me, I use 6 privacy screens (as featured in this picture) stacked on each other for daytime usage. Make sure when placing each privacy screen on each other that disruptive lines don't appear on the privacy screens. If lines appear when one privacy screen is placed on the other, try to switch the sides of the privacy screens until you find a combination of stacked privacy screens that do not cause squiggly lines. It will probably take a combination of several different brands of privacy screens to avoid the squiggly lines effect that is common with stacking privacy screens. Use kinesiology tape as desired to tape the stacked 2-6 privacy screens and secure the stacked privacy screens together on all 4 sides. It is important to note if I have to use a tablet at nighttime I add 2 loose extra privacy screens placed over the tablet (I rarely ever use devices at nighttime though).

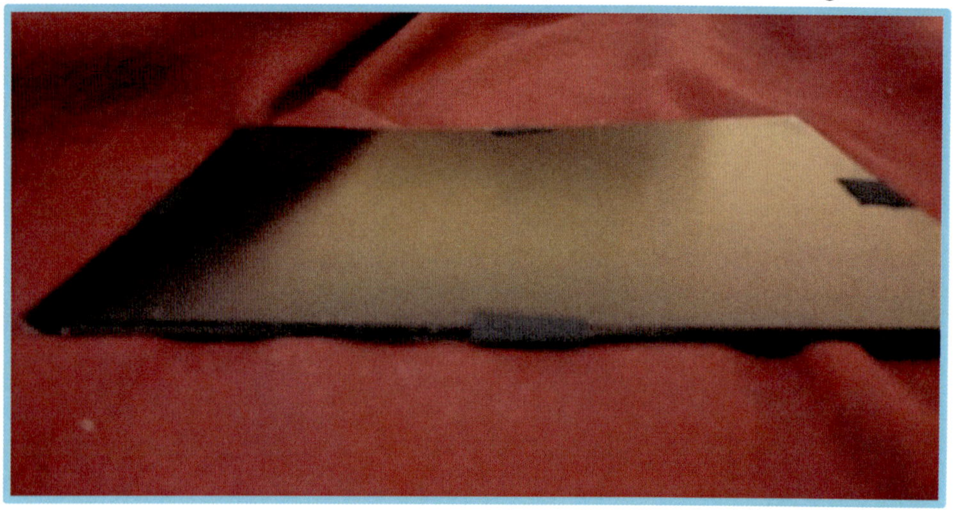

Step 2 Tablets: Place the 2-6 stacked privacy screens that were secured with kinesiology tape and place them over the tablet's screen. Now add kinesiology tape to all sides and secure the stacked privacy screens to the tablet. When you are securing the stacked privacy screens to the tablet, make sure to not cover up the speakers so that you can still hear the audio of the tablet. Not much kinesiology tape is needed to secure the 2-6 stacked privacy screens to the tablet (see picture below). I use 1-3 small kinesiology tapings on each side of the tablet to secure the stacked privacy screens to the tablet. Now that the tablet is secured with stacked privacy screens, the touch screen will probably not work and not register your fingerprints. I will address the solution to this problem in Step 3.

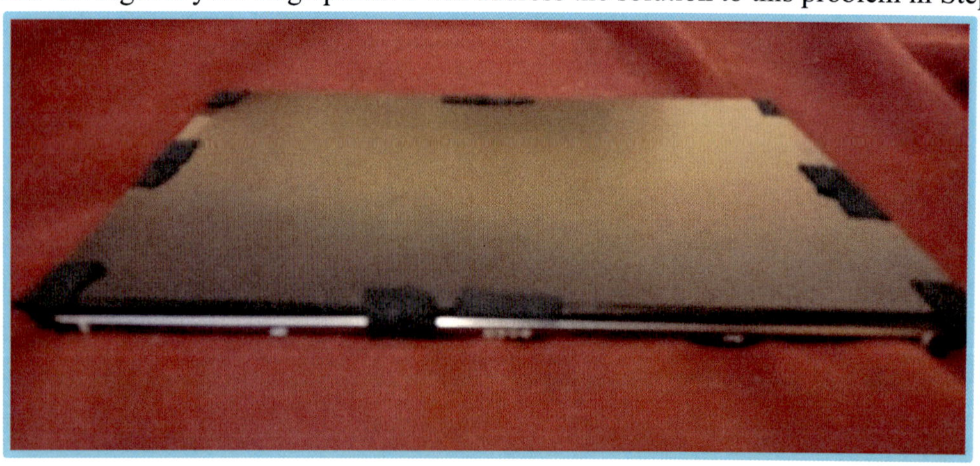

Step 3 Tablets: With the stacked privacy screens secured to the tablet, you will most likely be unable to use the touch screen. For this reason, a wireless "Amazon Basics Wireless Mouse with Nano Receiver" or a wired mouse with a wireless USB converter is needed. I used an Amazon Basics Mouse (wired or wireless) and an Amazon Basics Wireless USB converter called "USB Type C to USB 3.1 Gen1 Female Adapter". You can also use the Amazon Basics wireless USB converter for a wired mouse, as a USB mouse can plug into the wireless USB converter (the "USB Type C to USB 3.1 gen1 female Adapter").

-You will need a wireless mouse with a nano receiver (I.E Amazon Basics Mouse with nano receiver). Any wired or wireless mouse can also be used with the USB converter described below.

-You will need a "USB Type C to USB 3.1 gen1 female Adapter" (Amazon basics also makes this). This wireless USB converter is qute amazing: I discovered that it can be used for both a wireless mouse and a wired mouse.

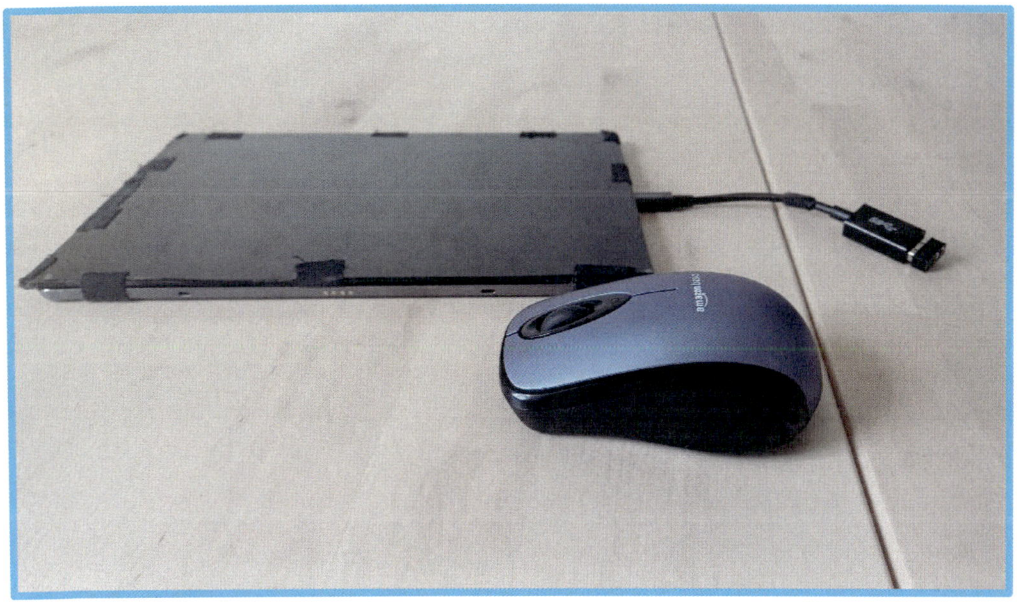

On the next page, I will show you how to apply the wireless nano receiver to the USB converter so that you can use a wireless mouse with a tablet. I will also show you how to plug in a wired mouse to the USB converter.

Step 3 Tablets Continued:

To plug in a wireless mouse to your wireless USB converter (the technical term is called a "USB Type C to USB 3.1 gen1 female Adapter"), all you must do is plug in the small nano receiver piece that was accompanied by the wireless mouse that you purchased into the USB converter. The nano receiver that accompanies a wireless mouse is small so be careful to not lose the nano receiver.

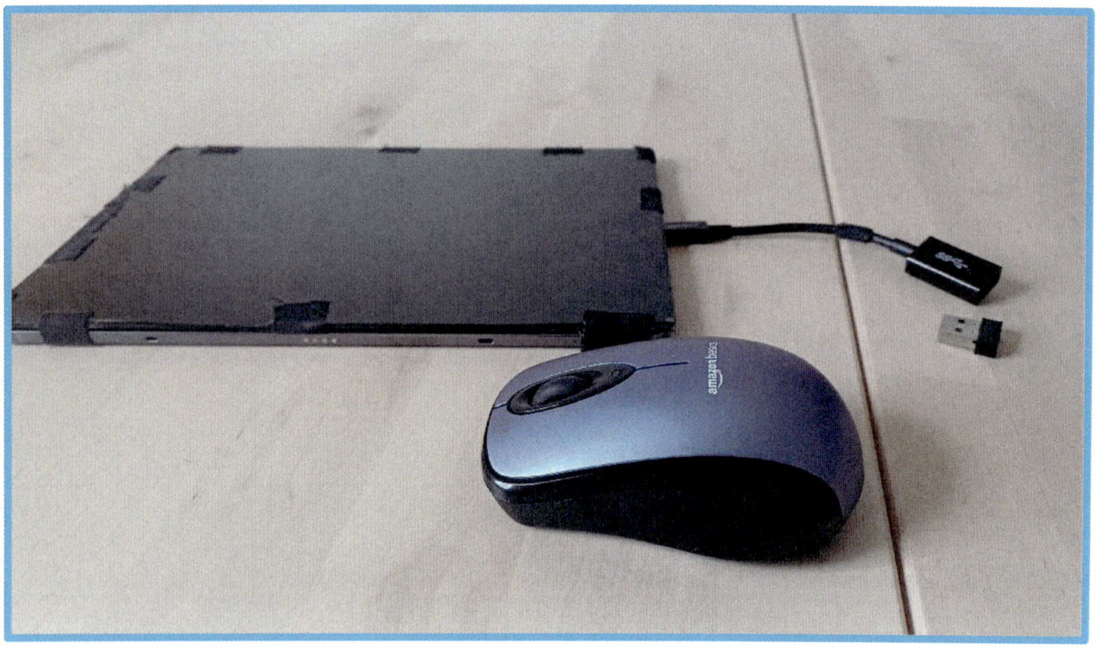

To use a wired mouse, simply plug in the USB wired mouse to the Wireless USB converter (the technical term is "USB Type C to USB 3.1 gen1 female Adapter") and it should work.

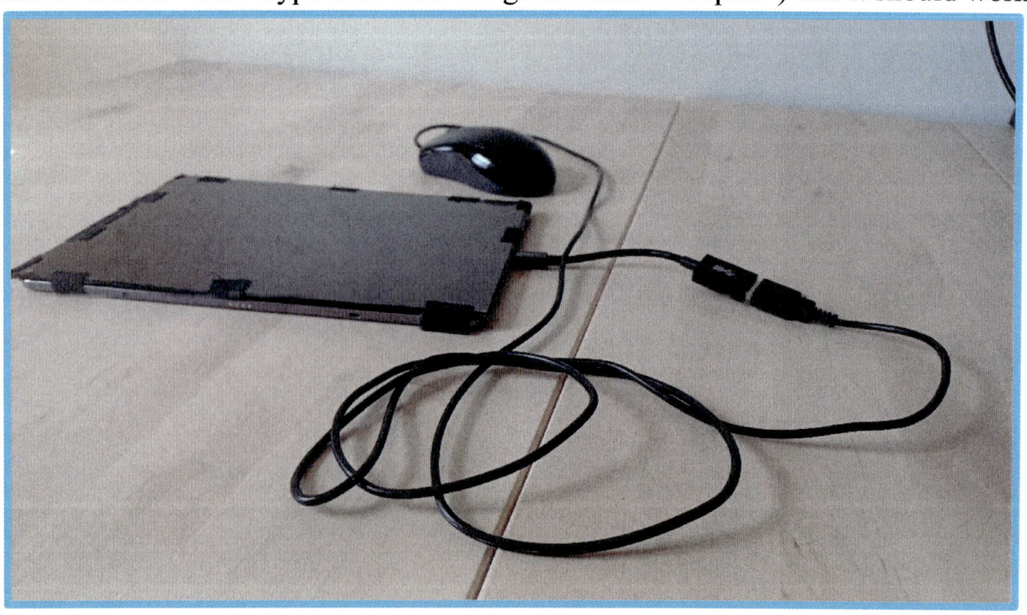

Step 4 Tablets: In step 4, I cover additional settings to reduce the amount of eye pain further.

Most tablets have a feature on settings to not only adjust the amount of brightness of the tablet, but also to enable "Eye Comfort Shields" or "Blue Light Reduction" settings. Through those settings you can customize how much you want to reduce blue light. I personally almost always use maximum 100% anti blue light reduction, to make it as easy on the eyes as possible. The only time when I adjust the anti-blue light feature to 50%-90% blue light reduction is when I am watching the tablet in daytime from far away (about 10 feet), and there is a detective show that I want to watch. When I use a tablet up-close, I always set the blue light reduction / eye comfort shield to 100% to reduce the amount of eye pain.

It is also important to note that not each tablet has the same blue light reduction effectiveness, and some tablets are harder on the eyes then others.

I personally use a refurbished galaxy tablet s6 as the screen has very effective blue light reduction settings and light reduction settings. Prior to using the galaxy tablet s6, I used the galaxy tablet s5e which also had great blue light reduction setting features. In my experience, the galaxy tablet amoled screens have been the easiest on the eyes for me with their effective and adjustable "eye comfort"/blue light reduction settings.

Step 5 Tablets: Placing the tablet on a tablet stand near a window with a lot of natural light is vital to reducing eye pain as much as possible from light sensitivity conditions. I actually rest the tablet on the tablet stand (although it sometimes falls down).
However, If I am using the tablet up close, I use the tablet while lying down near a large window to get the most possible natural light.

General Note: It is also important to note that I made the 6 privacy screens for the tablet from privacy screens that were created for desktop monitors (21.5 inches or larger). Desktop monitor privacy screens are good base privacy screens, as they are large, and they can be customized and used for smaller devices. Desktop privacy screens are good base privacy screens that can be customized and made smaller to be used for electronic devices such as tablets and laptops. Desktop privacy screens can also be used for small Televisions. I use privacy screens intended for desktop monitors on my television.

For example, I created many custom sized privacy screens for my tablet by using and cutting a larger privacy screen (I.E 21-inch to 32-inch) that was intended for desktop monitors at the workplace. This can help reduce the cost of using stacked privacy screens for tablets and other electronic devices.

Step 5 Tablets Continued: On sunny days, a wall divider with a bed linen of an ambient color may be needed to be able to see the contents of the tablet. You can also use a foamboard (instead of a wall divider) with a towel placed over it to control the amount of natural light that reaches the tablet's screen.

If it is too sunny, it may be impossible to see what is on the tablet. In the picture below, a large window is just to the left. Nearby the window, is a wall divider with a burgundy bed linen which can be moved in various angles to produce just the right amount of natural light needed. Alternatively, a foam board with a towel placed over it can be moved near the device to produce the right amount of natural light (see the picture on the next page, Pg. 16)

On sunny days, the goal is to be able to see the tablet's screen while still allowing a generous amount of natural light to reduce the amount of eye pain that may occur while using a tablet. For me, on sunny days, I may only use a wall divider or foamboard when the sun is facing directly at the window (which is only a couple of hours during the day). Careful adjustments and usages for the wall divider/foamboard will be needed on partly cloudy days and also on partly sunny days. On cloudy days, no wall divider/foamboard is needed for cloudy days, as cloudy days provide both natural light and screen visibility.

On cloudy days, I put my wall divider and foamboard away, and enjoy the natural light that it provides while still being able to see the contents on the tablet's screen. In the picture below, the tablet would be placed on the table on a tablet stand in the lower right corner of this picture. I also enjoy using my tablet while lying down near a window without a wall divider or foamboard for most times. The wall divider/foamboard may be helpful for those few hours during a day when the sun is facing directly at the window.

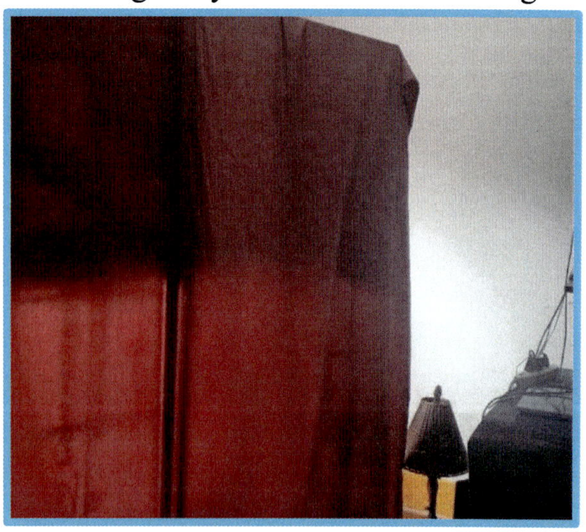

Step 5 Tablets Continued…: I will now demonstrate the usage of a foamboard instead of a wall divider (with a towel placed over it) to control the amount of natural light. This is a picture that I took which uses a foamboard with a towel placed over it to control the amount of natural light that goes to the electronic device's screen.
This picture has a television; however, if you are using a tablet, you would place the tablet on a tablet stand at a similar location on the table near where the television is.

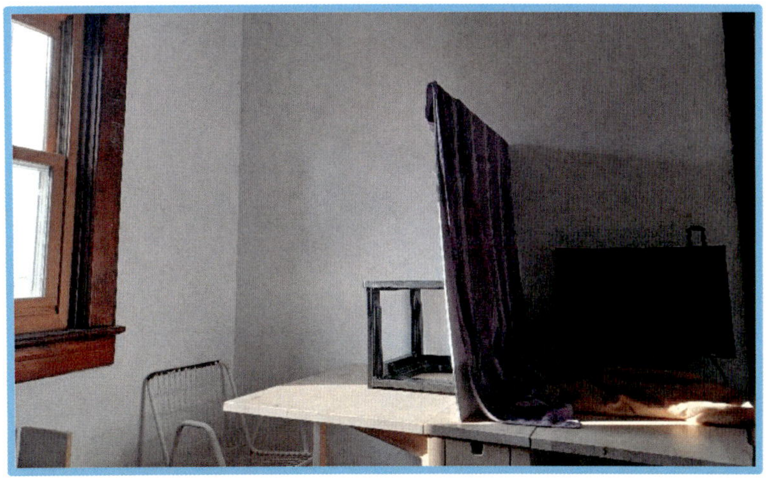

This is a picture of my current setup for using tablets. In my current setup, I do not need and do not use wall dividers or foamboards. Depending on what room you use, you may not need to use foamboards or wall dividers (even if it is sunny you may not need them).

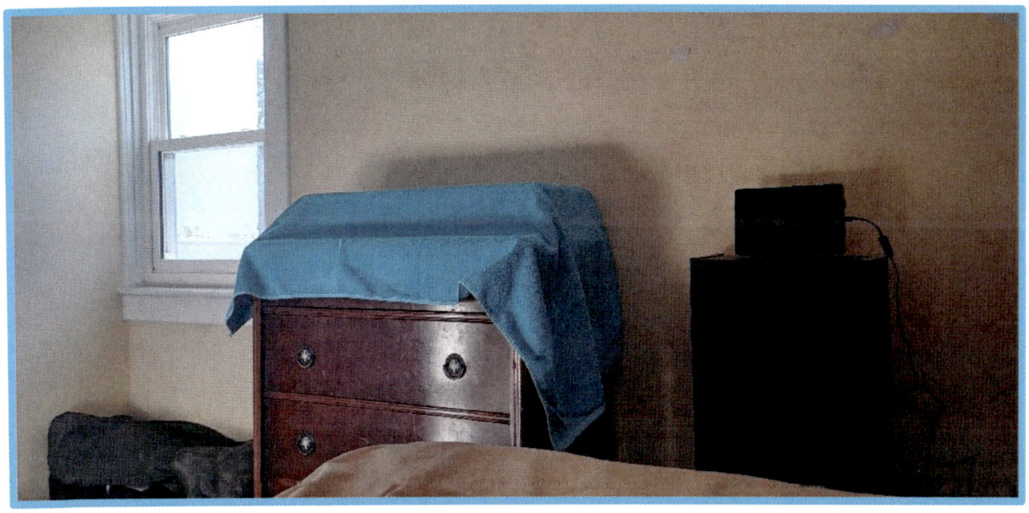

Note: you can raise the platform that the tablet stands on to make it easier on the eyes. By raising the height level of the tablet, you won't be looking directly at the tablet's screen (which can reduce eye pain). You can do this by adding textbooks (or a plastic container box) below the tablet & tablet stand. I personally rest my tablet on the tablet stand, rather then placing it on the tablet stand (the tablet often falls down on the textbook that it is standing on, but that is my preference).

Your Custom Tablet Settings

Use this blank space to document your customized techniques and solutions for reducing eye pain while using tablets (I.E How many stacked privacy screens are used & natural light settings or if you use wall dividers or foamboards: then what are your foamboard/wall divider settings). What are your tablet's "eye comfort shield" or "blue light reduction" settings.

Note: It is important to note that although I use 6 privacy screens placed on my tablet's screen, you may require less privacy screens.

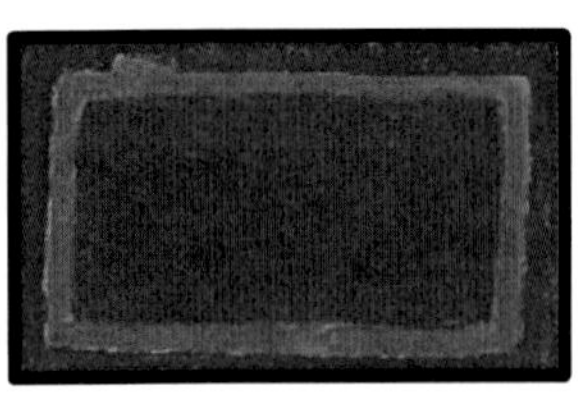

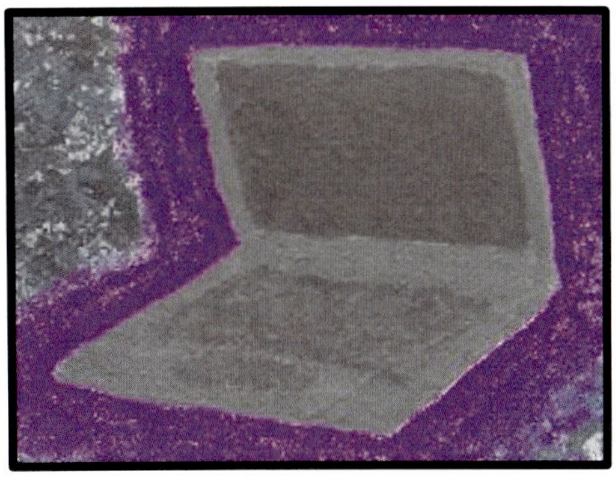

Chapter 3: Laptops

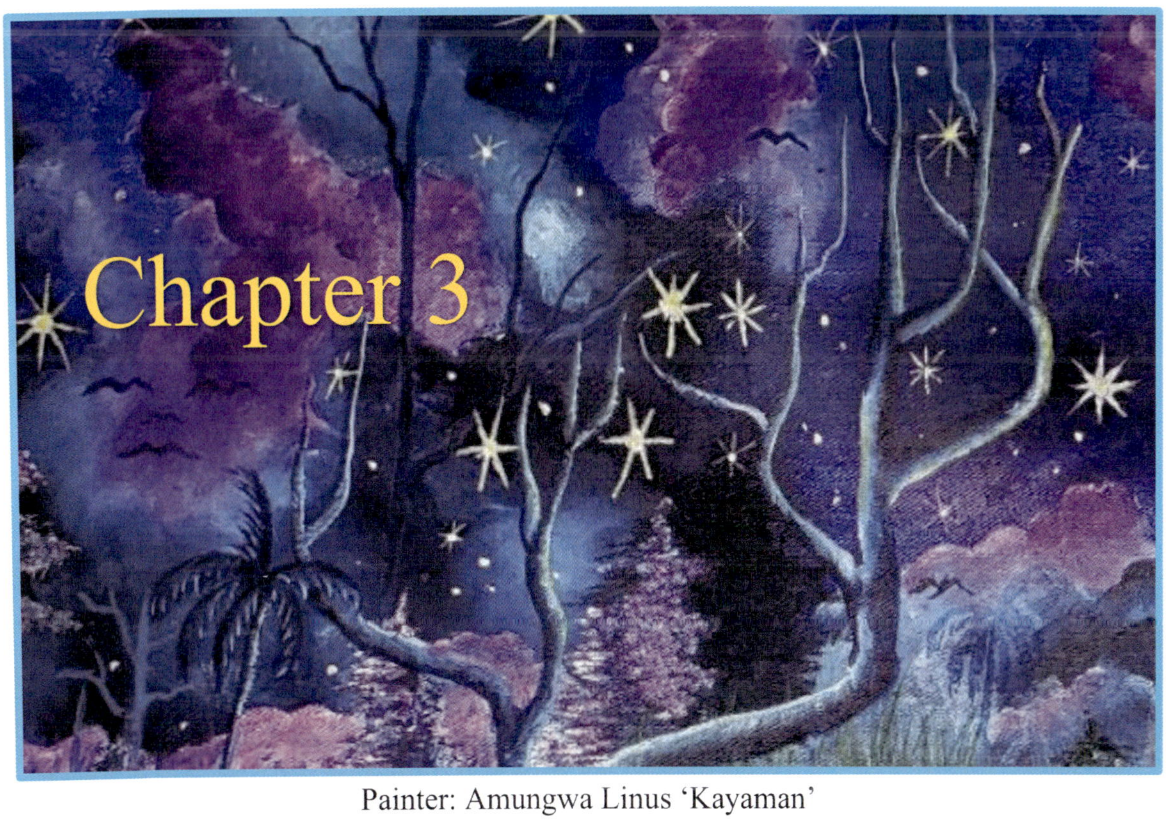

Painter: Amungwa Linus 'Kayaman'

Chapter 3 Laptops

A sudden accident which caused a chronic light sensitivity condition forced me to quit using laptops, until I found a solution.

Solution: It took 3 months to find a solution to enable me with the ability to use laptops. I tried dozens of glasses and none of them worked to reduce the eye pains that occurred while using laptops. I tried multiple blue light screens on my laptop and none of them worked to reduce the eye pains that occurred from using a laptop.

Fortunately, after several months of failed attempts, I thought of an idea to use multiple privacy screens stacked on my laptop by adding 1 or 2-5 privacy screens to my laptop (see Page 10 which explains "privacy screens"). I attempted the solution, and to my great relief, I was able to reduce the amount of eye pain that occurred from using laptops from significant to medium-mild. After developing this solution for my laptop, I was able to finish and publish my first book (*Goal Invention: The Mental Therapy, Sport, and Hobby*) and also type up my second book about cinema (which I wrote completely by hand during the 3 months of time while I was unable to use devices and had not yet thought of solutions).

It is important to point out though that there are times in the day when it is very sunny that I do not use privacy screens added on to the laptop. Sometimes on sunny days, I just use the laptop on minimum brightness & maximum blue light reduction settings / "eye comfort settings" (check your laptop's settings for this feature).

I was very relieved to finish my first project and get my second project's first edition finished. However, I was still dealing with medium eye pain throughout that process. Had it not been for my ambition to complete my projects, I would not have put myself through the eye pain. Because of the constant eye pain (albeit moderate instead of significant), I decided to experiment with natural light to reduce the amount of eye pain even more.

Natural Light + Solution: Unfortunately, it took me one year or so after the accident to use natural light to efficiently reduce the amount of eye pain that occurs while using laptops even more. I was so relieved and happy to finish my first book and also finish typing up the first edition of my second book (*How Cellphones Cropped, Distorted, and Visually Censored Cinema: Let's Save Cinema*) despite dealing with moderate eye pain throughout the process. I knew that I had to do something so that my eyes would not hurt as much for the second edition of the second book. (continued on the next page)

Chapter 3 Laptops

Natural Light + Solution Continued…: From that moment on, I decided to experiment with using the solution of using my laptop with stacked privacy screens near the window in the daytime with the aim of further reducing eye pain while using laptops.

I added 1 or 2-4 privacy screens stacked on my laptops' screens in the middle of the day near the window, and to my great relief I was able to reduce the amount of eye pain that occurred from using laptops. I was very relieved that with natural light, in combination with the solution of stacked privacy screens, I was able to reduce the amount of eye pain and eye strains that occurred from using laptops. It is important to point out that I did not use privacy screens on the laptop if it was very sunny.

A difficult reality with laptop and computer-work for individuals with chronic light sensitivity conditions, is that eye pain is very difficult to avoid. Even with natural light and stacked privacy screens, it is very difficult to use computers and laptops in a professional setting on a 9am – 5pm fulltime basis. I would not use laptops or computers for anything other than to type my life's works. I enjoy using my laptop while near a window with a lot of natural light to further reduce the amount of eye pain that occurs from using laptops.

The typing and computer experience is stressful and often can be painful for individuals with light sensitivity conditions, but with solutions and techniques, written projects may be able to be achieved with milder amounts of eye pain.
It is important to note that written projects for individuals with light sensitivity conditions take patience and take much longer to complete, as a lot of time involves resting the eyes for days and potentially weeks or months at a time. I lost count of the amount of times I took days, weeks, and even month-long breaks from using laptops (or any device at all) for my eye pain to subside. In some cases it took several months for the eye pain and eye strains to subside. After I completed my first two books, I switched to writing short books so that I could reduce the amount of eye pain that I would experience from using laptops.

Light sensitivity and computer/laptop work is difficult and takes patience for individuals with chronic light sensitivity conditions. I try to use laptops as little as possible. For example, following my first book, I handwrote the first editions of all my books on physical notebooks before typing them to a word document and I also completed most of my edits on physical printouts prior to typing the edits to Word.

Chapter 3 Laptops: The Setup Process

Step 1: For laptops, kinesiology tape is not necessarily needed, but the same method of making custom fitted stacked privacy screens with kinesiology tape can be done. For me, I use 1 or 2-6 loose stacked privacy screens without kinesiology tape for laptops, so that I can easily adjust how many privacy screens I need. Kinesiology tape is not needed for laptops as the privacy screens can rest on the base of the laptop.
In the picture below, no kinesiology tape is used.
If it is very sunny and I am near a window, I may not use any privacy screens at all.
It is important to note that I do all my computer work on laptops, as the smaller screens of laptops are much easier on the eyes then desktop monitors.

Step 2: Almost all laptops now have a feature on settings to not only adjust the amount of brightness of the laptop, but also to enable "Eye Comfort Shields" or "Blue Light Reduction" settings. Through that setting you can customize how much you want to reduce blue light on your laptop. It is important to note that not each laptop has the same blue light reduction effectiveness, and some laptops cause more eye pain then others.

Step 3: Placing the laptop on a table near a window with a lot of natural light is vital to reducing eye pain as much as possible from light sensitivity conditions. My laptop in the picture below is only a few meters away from a large window which provides good natural light (this is where I often do laptop work). In addition, I enjoy using my laptops while lying down near a window with natural light in order to reduce eye pain.

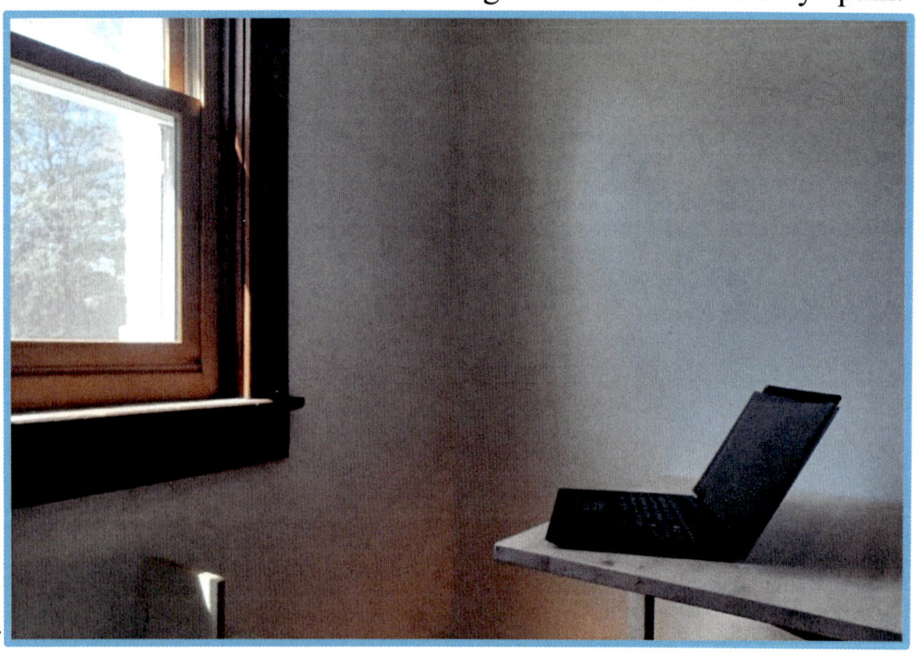

Chapter 3 Laptops: The Setup Process Continued...

This is an example of using privacy screens loosely placed over a laptop. This is my favorite method of using privacy screens for laptops because it is very easy to customize the amount of privacy screens that are being used. If I am near a window and it is very sunny and I can't see the contents on the laptop's screen, I will remove the privacy screens. Sometimes, I will not use privacy screens at all (if it is sunny and I am near a window). If you are near a window on a sunny day, you may not need privacy screens.

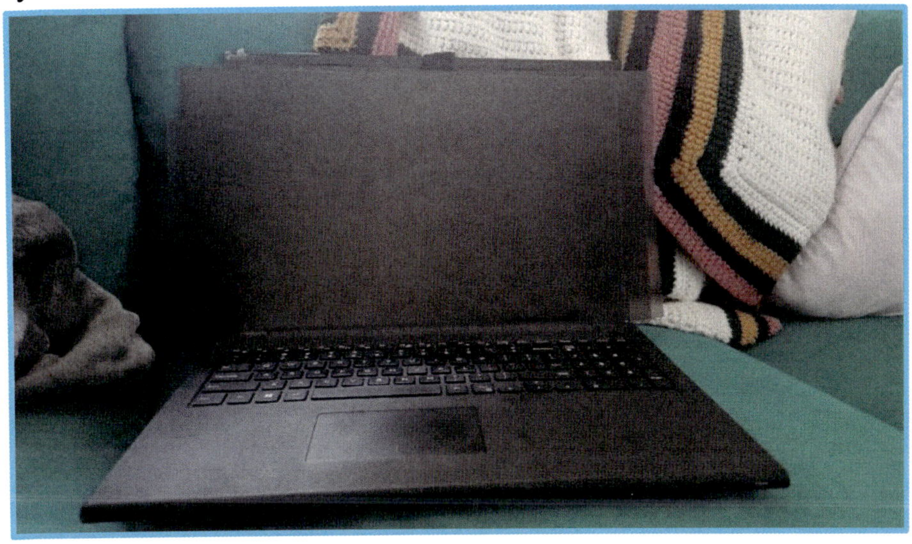

This is an example of applying privacy screens directly to a laptop with kinesiology tape.

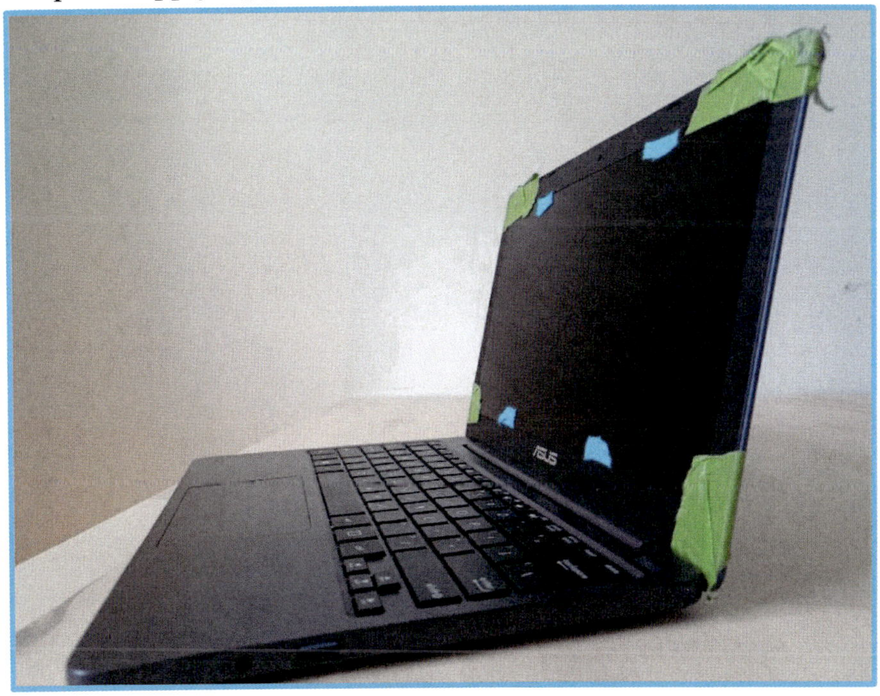

Chapter 3 Laptops: The Setup Process Continued...

For individuals with chronic light sensitivity conditions, harnessing the natural light from a nearby window is vital towards reducing the amount of eye pain and eye strains that occur from using laptops.

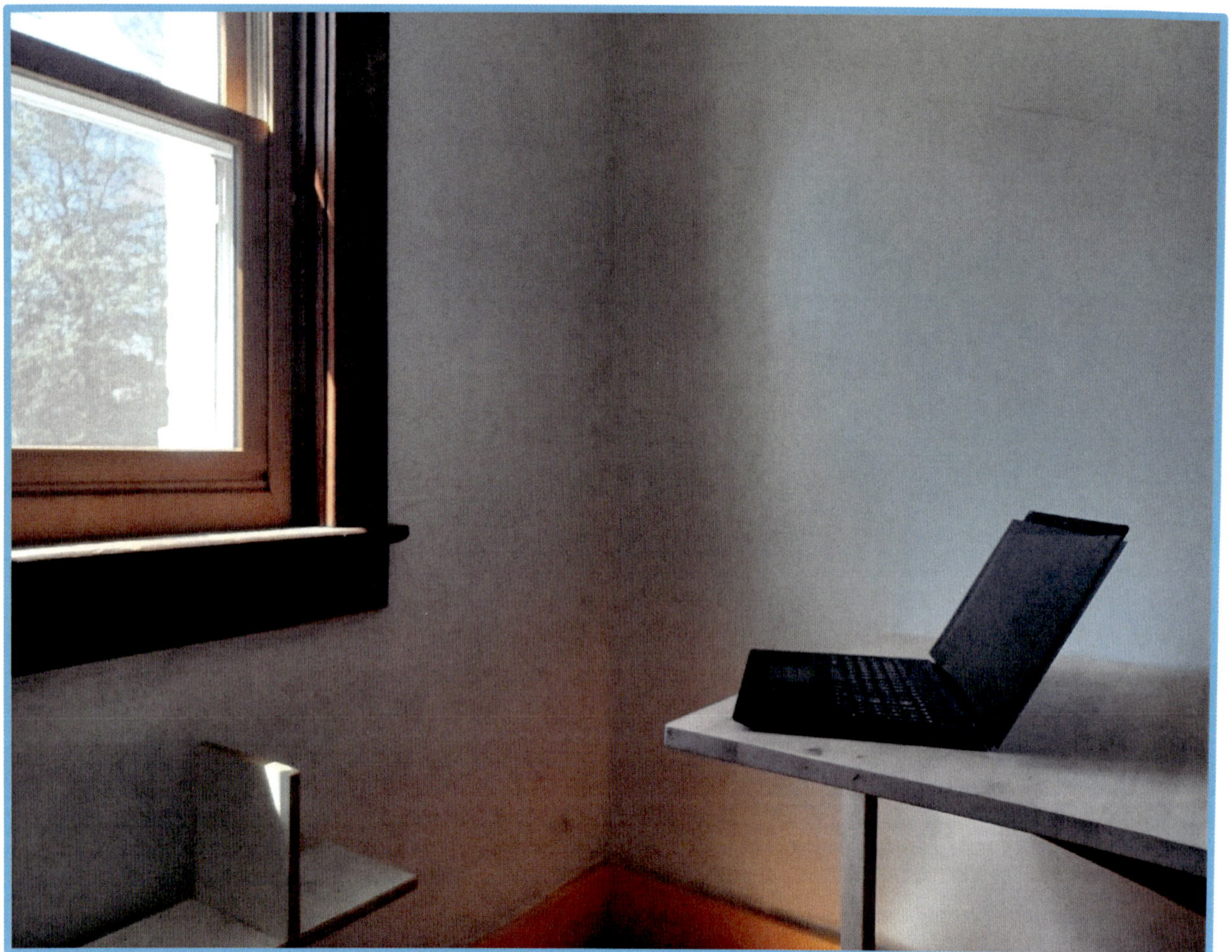

I only use laptops on sunny days near a window. If it is cloudy or it is evening-nighttime, I put away the laptop so that I can reduce the amount of eye pain and eye strains that may occur.

It is important to note that I do all my computer work on laptops, as the smaller screens of laptops are much easier on the eyes then desktop monitors.

Your Custom Laptop Settings

Use this blank space to document your customized techniques and solutions for reducing eye pain while using laptops (I.E How many stacked privacy screens or loose privacy screens are used & what are your natural light settings). If you used wall dividers or foamboards: then what are your foamboard/wall divider settings. What are your laptop's "eye comfort shield" or "blue light reduction" settings.

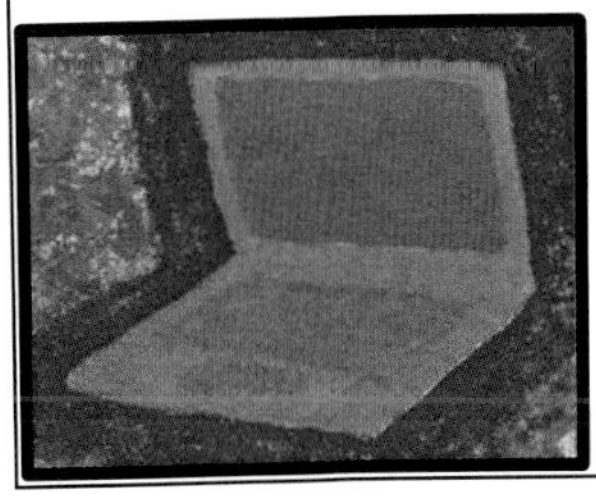

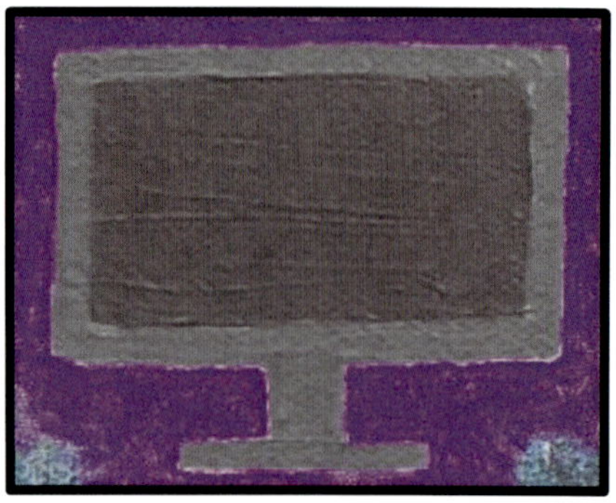

Chapter 4: Televisions & Desktop Monitors

Note: It is important to note that while I include desktop monitors prominently in this chapter, I do all my computer work on laptops. The smaller screens of laptops are much easier on the eyes then desktop monitors. For computer work, laptops are easier on the eyes than desktop monitors.

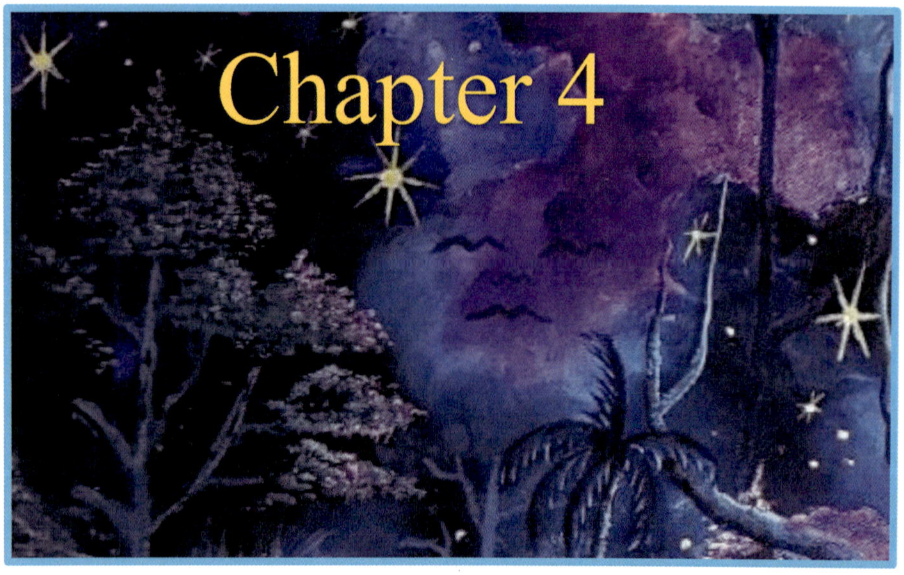

Painter: Amungwa Linus 'Kayaman'

Chapter 4 TVs and Monitors

Origins: A sudden accident occurred which caused a chronic light sensitivity condition. I quit using televisions and monitors for a total of 4 months until I developed a solution to enable me to use televisions and desktop monitors without strong eye pain occurring.

Solution: It took about 4 months to find a solution to enable me to watch televisions and desktop monitors. I tried watching televisions and desktop monitors with dozens of different anti-blue light glasses without any success in reducing the amount of eye pain that occurred. I tried many anti-blue light screens placed on my television and desktop monitor with no success, as the eye pain that occurred from the light sensitivity condition was too significant for me to use televisions and desktop monitors.

After several months of failing attempts to reduce eye pain and eye strains while using televisions and desktop monitors, I thought of a solution. The solution involved the application of multiple (6-7) privacy screens stacked to my television and desktop monitors with kinesiology tape (see Pg. 10 for details about privacy screens).
I attempted the solution of stacking 6 privacy screens together and placing them on a 21-inch television monitor, and fortunately the amount of eye pains and strains that I experienced were significantly reduced. Finally, 4 months after the small sudden accident, I was able to watch televisions and monitors (albeit with limited visibility and limited usage) without causing significant eye pain. While the eye pain was reduced significantly, it was not until a year after the accident, that I discovered how to implement natural light to reduce eye pains that occur while using televisions/monitors even more.

Solution + Natural Light: I was so relieved and happy to be able to use and watch televisions and desktop monitors again. The solution of adding 6-7 privacy screens onto the TV/Monitor reduced the eye pain from using TVs and desktop monitors. However, it took a year for me to make the decision to experiment with natural light while using the TVs and monitors to reduce eye pains and strains even more. **(continued on the next page)**

Chapter 4 TVs and Monitors Continued...

Solution + Natural Light Continued...: I attempted to use the 21-inch TV monitor with 6-7 stacked privacy screens placed on the TV/Monitor and then I placed the TV/Monitor on a table near a window in daytime. I used Kinesiology tape to tape the privacy screens together, and I then used Kinesiology tape to secure the stacked privacy screens over the Television monitor. The solution involving natural light was created with the aim of reducing eye pain and eye strains that occur while using televisions and monitors. Fortunately, the combination of stacked privacy screens and natural light worked great, and the techniques reduced the amount of eye pain and strains that occurred from using televisions/monitors. To this day, I use almost all of my screen time in the daytime near a window with the aid of natural light to reduce the amount of eye pain that occurs.

The only issue of natural light that occurred with applying the solution of natural light was the varying amounts of natural light of different weather days. For cloudy days, the natural light through the window was sufficient and constant and I could still see the contents of the television/monitor screen. At some times during sunny days, there was too much natural light to see the screen, so I used a wall divider in front of the window with a maroon bed linen sheet placed over the wall divider. I later realized that a foamboard with a towel placed over the foamboard could be used instead of a wall divider to control the amount of natural light that reaches a television monitor or desktop monitor.

The wall divider/foamboard with the bed sheet/towel (placed over) on top worked great, as I was able to customize the amount of natural light that I needed in order to reduce the amount of eye pain and eye strains that occurred. The walldivider/foamboard provided me with the ability to customize how much natural light reaches the television/monitor. On sunny days and partly cloudy days, I move and adjust the wall divider/foamboard with the sheet/towel (placed over the foamboard or wall divider) to adjust the amount of natural light that reaches the television/desktop monitor.

Chapter 4 TVs and Monitors Continued...

Solution + Natural Light Continued...: The goal of using wall dividers/foamboards is to be able to see the contents that appear on the television/monitor screen, but also reduce the amount of eye strains and eye pain that occur from watching TVs/Monitors. It is important to note however on sunny days, that I do not use wall dividers/foamboards on all the time for Televisions/Monitors. For example, on sunny days, in the morning until 2pm, I use my TV/Desktop Monitor without using a wall divider or a foamboard. Depending on where the sun is and where your windows are, you may not need to use a wall divider or a foam board. On sunny days, I particularly only use the wall divider/foamboard in the afternoon when the sun is facing directly at my windows (in order to control the amount of natural light).

The goal is to get as much possible natural light to your TV/Monitor while still being able to see the contents of the screen on the television/desktop monitor. On both sunny days and cloudy days, I enjoy using my Television/Monitor without a wall divider/foamboard from the morning to 2pm and also during other parts of the afternoon when the sun is not beaming at the window. Again, a wall divider or a foamboard may only be needed when the sun is facing directly at the window.

* TV and Monitor Privacy Screen Squiggly/Wavy Line Problem

I added this paragraph to note that when you stack privacy screens on one another, you may see squiggly/wavy lines appear on the privacy screens. This problem may be fixed by switching the side of the privacy screens one by one to the other side until a combination occurs that produces no squiggly/wavy lines. For my stacked privacy screens which I placed on my Television Monitor, I used a combination of desktop monitor privacy screens (from various companies) and I switched the privacy screens to the other side as necessary until I found a stacked combination of privacy screens (secured together by kinesiology tape) that did not produce squiggly/wavy lines on the privacy screens.

Chapter 4 TVs and Monitors - The Setup Process

Step 1: Custom fit your privacy screens to the desired size of your TV's/Desktop Monitor's screen size and pick your desired amount of privacy screens stacked on each other (from 2-7) depending on preference. For me, I use 6-7 privacy screens stacked on each other for daytime usage of privacy screens. Make sure when placing each privacy screen on each other that disruptive lines don't appear. If squiggly lines/waves appear when one privacy screen is placed on the other, try to switch the sides of the privacy screens until you find a combination of stacked privacy screens that do not cause squiggly lines. It will probably take a combination of several different brands of privacy screens to avoid the squiggly lines effect that is common with stacking privacy screens. Use kinesiology tape as desired to tape the stacked 2-7 privacy screens and secure them together on all 4 sides (see picture below).

In the picture below, there are six or seven 21.5-inch privacy screens that are taped together (on the outside) on all four sides with kinesiology tape. Only a few small kinesiology tapes are needed on each side of the stacked privacy screens to secure the group of privacy screens.
I only use TVs/Monitors in the daytime in order to use natural light to help reduce eye pain. I do not use or look at any devices' screens at evening-nighttime, as there is no natural light available at that time to reduce the amount of eye pain that occurs from watching devices' screens.
Note: It is important to note that I use 6 or 7 privacy screens placed on my TV/Desktop Monitor, yet you may require less privacy screens placed on your TV/Monitor (I.E 3-5 privacy screens).

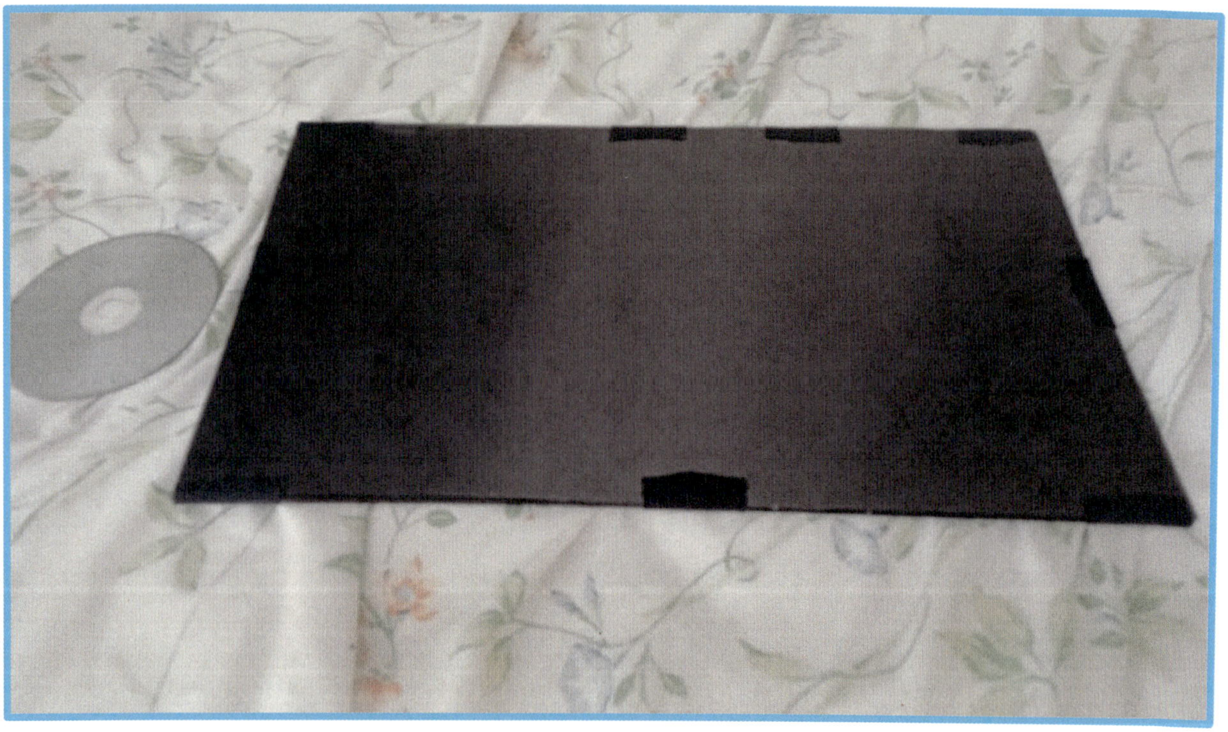

Step 2: Place the 2-7 stacked privacy screens that were secured with kinesiology tape and place it over the Television/Desktop Monitor's screen. Now add kinesiology tape to all sides of the TV/Monitor and secure the stacked privacy screens to the TV/Monitor. A lot of kinesiology tape is needed to secure the 2-7 stacked privacy screens to the TV/Monitor (as seen in the picture below) as the larger sized privacy screens weigh more (see in the picture below, the 21.5-inch privacy screens). I use entire full-length strips of kinesiology tape on all four sides to secure the stacked privacy screens to the TV/Desktop Monitor. It will require multiple full-length strips of kinesiology tape to secure the 2-7 stacked privacy screens to the TV/Monitor. Using smaller sized 21.5 – 27-inch televisions is easier on the eyes, and also required, as the largest desktop monitor privacy screens are within the 21 – 32-inch range.
The television featured in the picture below is 21 inches in size. Now that the Television/Desktop Monitor is secured with stacked privacy screens, there are few additional techniques to address.

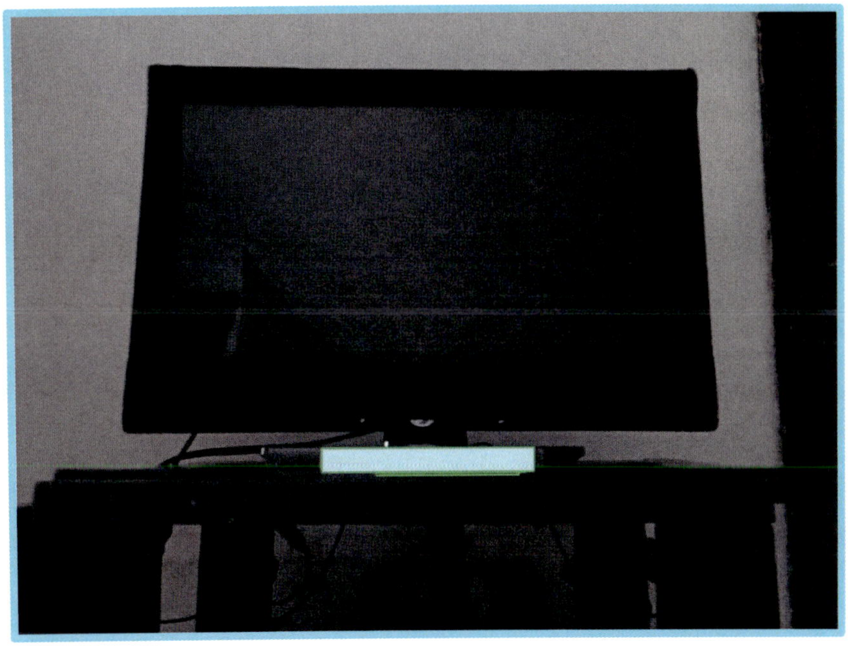

Note: you can raise the platform that the Television stands on to make it easier on the eyes. By raising the height level of the Television, you won't be looking directly at the Television's screen (which can reduce eye pain). You can do this by adding textbooks (or a plastic container box) below the Television. I am using a plastic container box in the picture above.

When there is not enough natural light to use a Television/Desktop Monitor (I.E evening or nighttime), I listen to audiobooks or listen (without watching) to shows on my tablet from evening to nighttime. To this day, it is difficult to adjust to this lifestyle decision, but it helps to reduce the amount of eye pain and eye strains that I experience. If there is a sport game that occurs at nighttime, I will not watch the game and I will watch it on replay in the natural light another day.

Step 3: In Step 3, I cover additional settings to reduce the amount of eye pain further.

Some TVs and Desktop monitors have a feature on settings to not only adjust the amount of brightness of the Television/Desktop Monitor, but also to enable "Eye Comfort Shields" or "Blue Light Reduction" settings. Through that setting you can customize how much you want to reduce blue light. It is also important to note that not each TV/Monitor has the same blue light reduction effectiveness, and some TVs/Monitors cause more eye pain than others.

Step 4: Placing the Television/Desktop Monitor on a table near a window with a lot of natural light is vital to reducing eye pain as much as possible from light sensitivity conditions (as seen in the picture below). My television in the picture is a few meters from a large window which provides great natural light. Also, it is important to note that I add a raised platform on top of the table, so that the TV is higher. I also add a DVD box to tilt the TV slightly upwards so that I can reduce the amount of eye pain that occurs. This is due to the effect of privacy screens: if you are not looking directly at privacy screens, there is a darkening effect. The addition of a raised platform box on the table and a DVD box underneath the TV to tilt the TV back (slightly) helps to release some of the pressure and prevents looking at the TV/Monitor directly head on. When a TV/Monitor is slightly tilted upward, you can still see the screen, but you also reduce the amount of eye pain that may occur while using a TV/Monitor. These two subtle adjustments help to reduce the amount of eye pain that occurs while using televisions and desktop monitors. Textbooks can also be used to place under the TV/Monitor to raise the TV/Monitor. When I raise my television higher with stacks of textbooks (under the TV), I notice that less eye pain occurs.

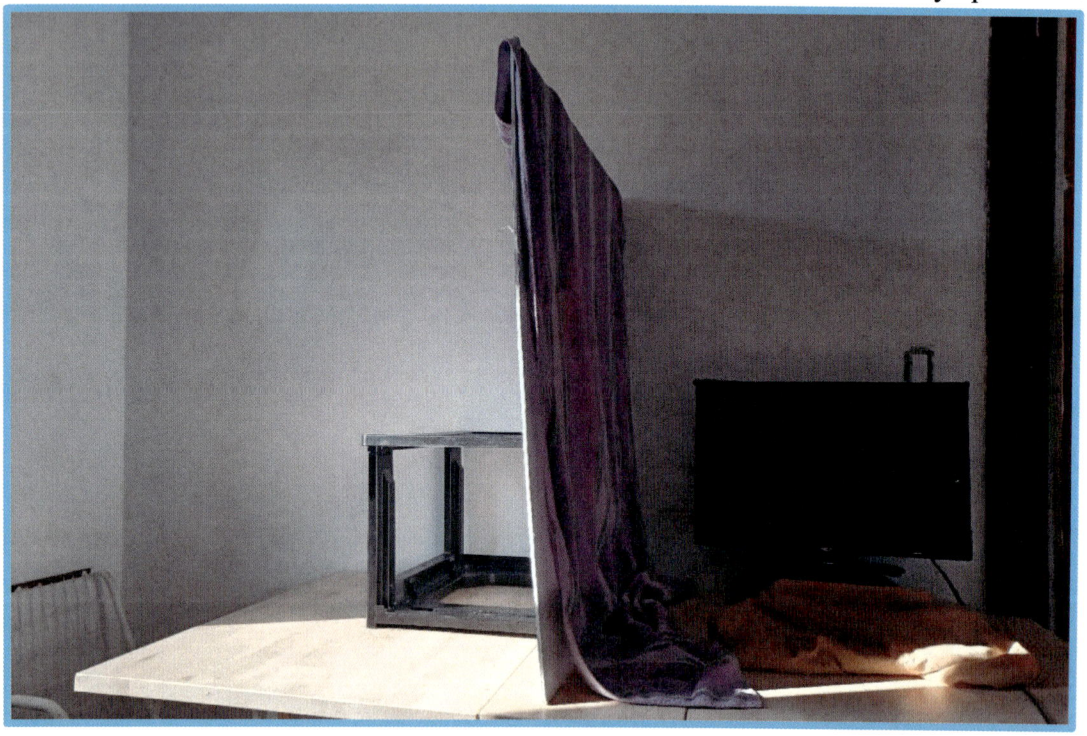

Step 5: On sunny days, a wall divider or a foamboard with a bed linen/towel of an ambient color may be needed to be able to see the contents of the Television/Desktop Monitor. If it is too sunny, it may be impossible to see what is on the TV/Monitor's screen. In the picture below, a large window is just to the left. Nearby the window, is a wall divider with a burgundy bed linen sheet which can be moved in various angles to produce just the right amount of natural light needed. On sunny days, the goal is to be able to see the TV/Monitor while still allowing a generous amount of natural light to reach the room that you are in (in order to reduce the amount of eye pain that may occur while using TVs/Monitors). On sunny days, I only use a wall divider or a foamboard (with a bedsheet/towel placed over it) when the sun is facing directly at the window (which is only a couple of hours).Careful adjustments and usages for the wall divider or foamboard will be needed on partly cloudy days. Fortunately, no wall divider or foamboard is needed for cloudy days, as cloudy days provide both natural light and screen visibility. On cloudy days, I put my wall divider/foamboard away, and enjoy the natural light that it provides while still being able to see the contents on the TV/Monitor.

The Usage of a Wall Divider to Control Natural Light

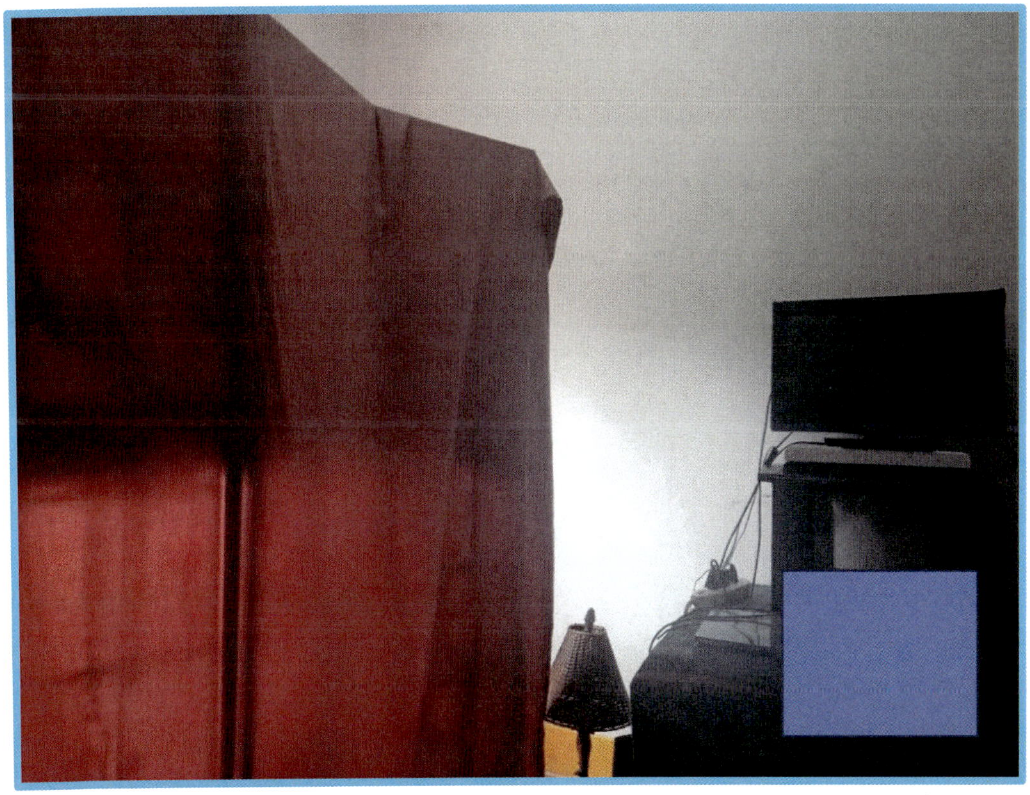

The above picture illustrates the usage of a wall divider to control the amount of natural light that reaches a Television / Desktop Monitor.

Step 5 Continued...: The picture below is an example of the usage of a foamboard (instead of a wall divider) that is placed between the window and the TV/Monitor (this controls how much natural light reaches the TV/Monitor's screen). A large foamboard should be able to be purchased at an arts and crafts store or online. Notice the usage of a large window that creates excellent natural light. The foamboard is my personal favorite.

The Usage of a Foamboard to Control Natural Light

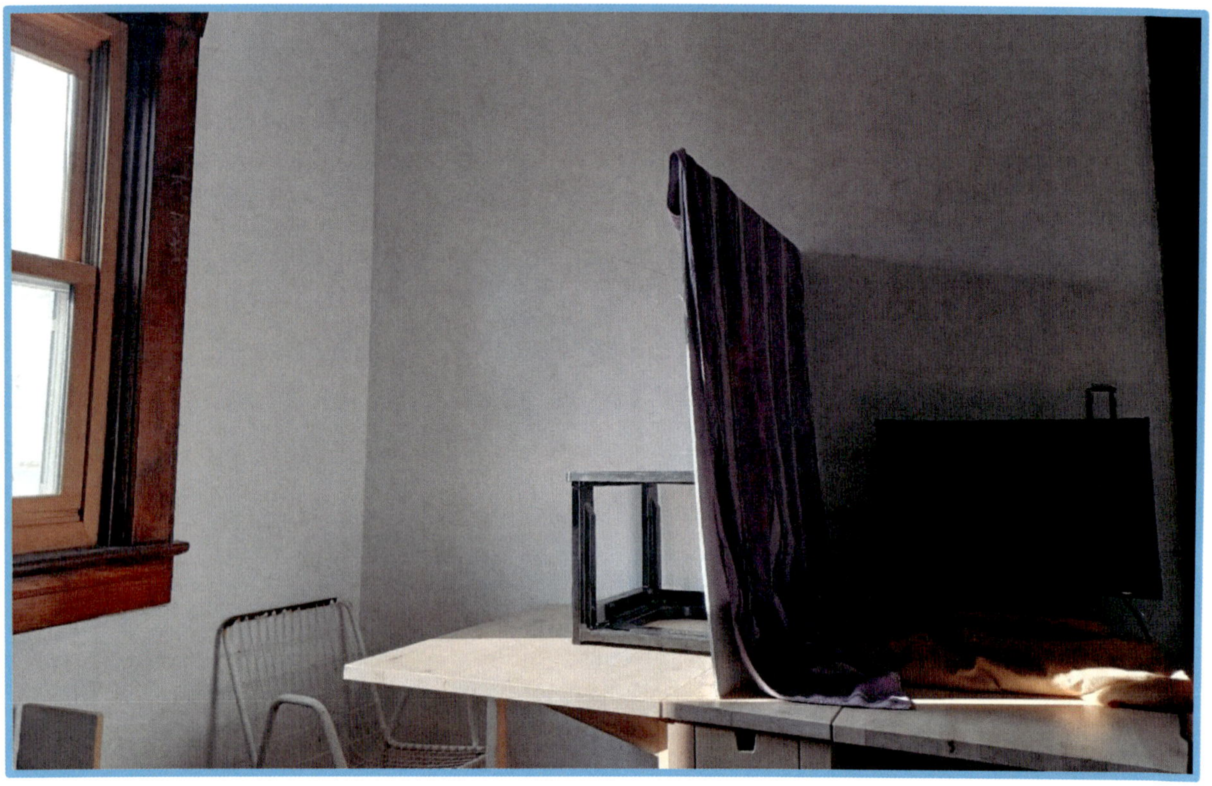

Note: In this picture, I am using textbooks below the television to raise the viewing height of the TV, so that I don't look directly straight on at the television's screen (this is easier on the eyes).

The above picture illustrates the usage of a foamboard to control the amount of natural light that reaches a Television/Desktop Monitor. Controlling the amount of natural light that reaches a TV/Monitor screen, allows you to better be able to see the contents on the TV/Monitor's screen. I discovered the usage of the foamboard this past year, and it is now my go to method for controlling natural light. I still feel that a wall divider may be the right option for some individuals. A towel is needed to be placed over the foamboard to further intensify the effectiveness of controlling the amount of natural light that reaches the screen.

The goal is to use as much natural light that is needed to reduce eye pain while also being able to see the contents of the television or desktop monitor's screen.

Your Custom Television / Desktop Monitor Settings

Use this blank space to document your customized techniques and solutions for reducing eye pain while using Televisions/Monitors (I.E How many stacked privacy screens are used & natural light settings. What are your wall divider and foamboard settings). What are your Television/Monitor's "eye comfort shield" or "blue light reduction" settings (most TV's do not have such features).

Note: Although I use 6-7 privacy screens placed on my Television/Desktop Monitor's screen, you may require less privacy screens placed on your TV/Monitor's screen (I.E 3-5 privacy screens).

Additional Note: While I include desktop monitors prominently in this chapter, I do all my computer work on laptops (the smaller screens of laptops are easier on the eyes than monitors).

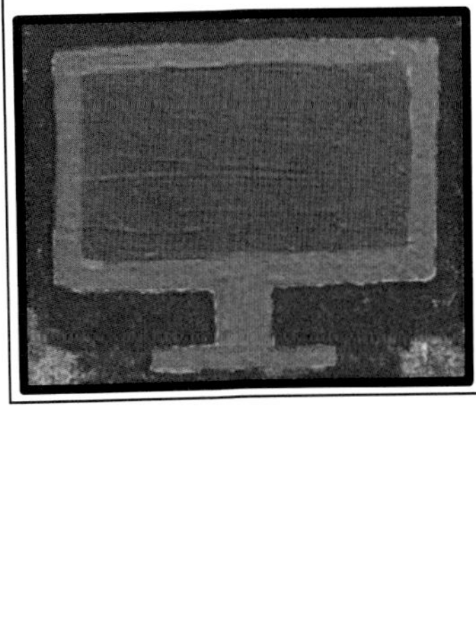

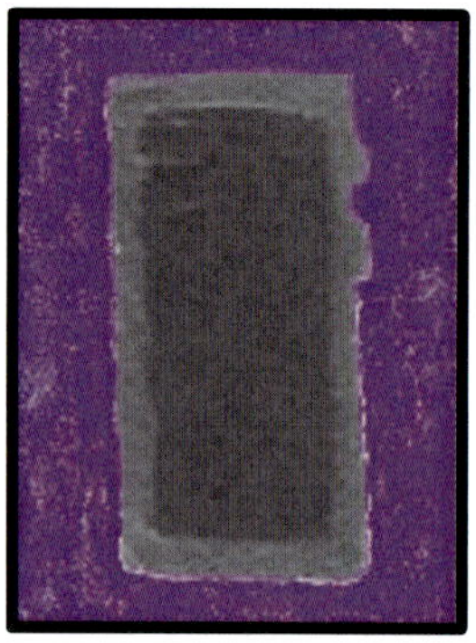

Chapter 5:

Cellphones

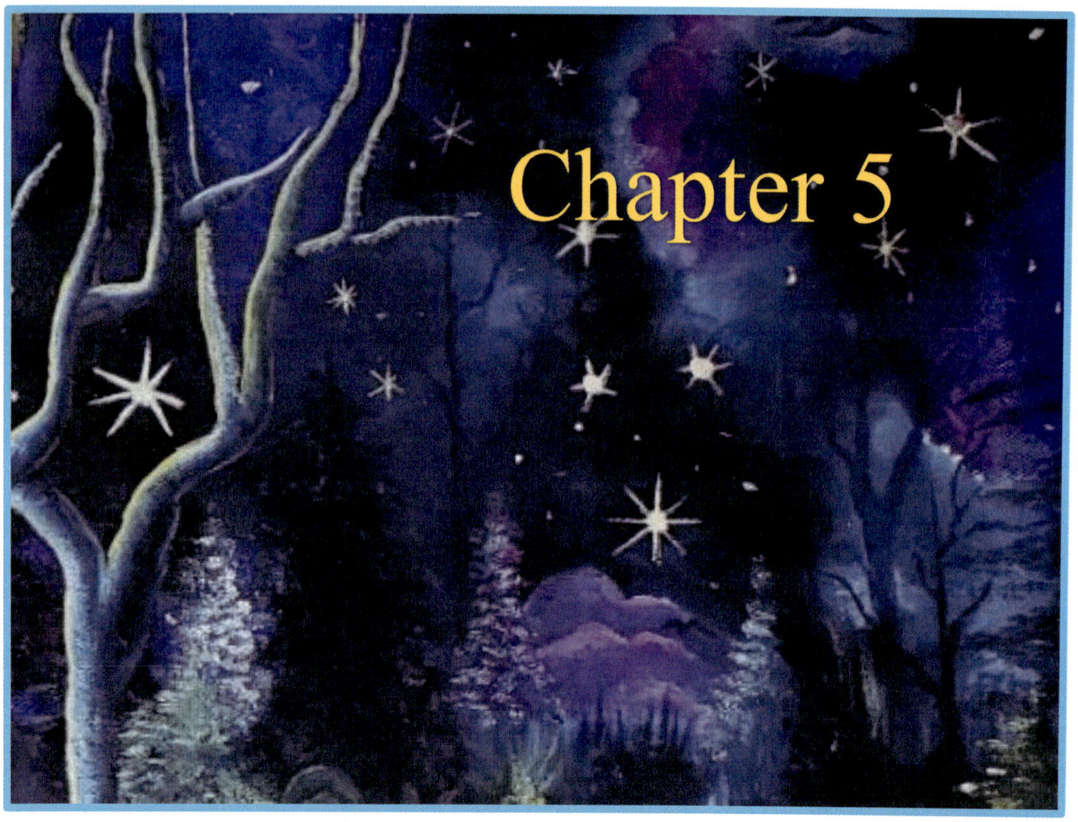

Painter: Amungwa Linus 'Kayaman'

Chapter 5 Cellphones:

The sudden accident, which caused a chronic light sensitivity condition, forced me to quit cellphones for 4 months.

Solution: It took 4 months to find a solution to enable me to use cellphones (albeit with limited usage). I tried dozens of anti-blue light glasses, and nothing worked to reduce eye pain while using cellphones. I tried multiple anti-blue light screens placed on my cellphone and that also failed to reduce eye pains while using cellphones.
Fortunately, I thought of a solution to try multiple privacy screens stacked on my cellphone (see Page 10 for details about privacy screens). I used 2-3 privacy screens and stacked the privacy screens on my cellphone, and the eye pain that I experienced from using cellphones was reduced. It was great that the solution worked to enable me to use cellphones in a limited capacity. It is important to note that companies sell custom fitted privacy screens for cellphones (just search your cellphone's name + "privacy screen" and you will find custom fitted privacy screens available to purchase on online retailers).

Solution + Natural Light: It would take a year after the injuries to my eyes until I experimented with natural light to reduce the amount of eye pain that occurs while using cellphones. I used my cellphone with 1-3 privacy screens stacked on the cellphone near a window in daytime, and I was happy that it caused even less pain to the eyes. To this day, I use my cellphone and all devices almost exclusively in the daytime near a window in order to cause less eye pain from using devices. It is important to note however that due to chronic light sensitivity induced from a small accident, I had to quit all forms of mobile gaming including games on the phone. It is also important to note that I use cellphones for only 10 or 30 minutes a day or so.

Step 1: Applying privacy screens to cellphones is the simplest of all devices. This is because privacy screens are popular for cellphones. Simply search for privacy screens that are made for your exact cellphone brand, and they will be custom fitted to fit your cellphone. The unfortunate reality of cellphones is that there can probably only be 2-3 privacy screens (max) placed on a cellphone before the cellphone's finger censor does not work. I use 1-3 privacy screens stacked on my cellphone. Due to the touch screen being an important part of the cellphone experience, (probably) only a maximum of 2-3 privacy screens can be applied to a cellphone's screen at a time (and this helps to reduce eye pain while using cellphones).

Chapter 5 Cellphones:

Step 2: After 1-3 custom privacy screens are applied to your cellphone's screen, it is vital to use the cellphone near windows with good natural light and primarily in the daytime. I almost always use my cellphone lying down on the ground near a window with a lot of natural light in the daytime. It is important to note that I do not use cellphones for more then 10-30 minutes a day. I usually only apply two privacy screens to the cellphone which I use, as I rarely ever use the cellphone (and I only use the cellphone in the natural light near a window).

Step 3: Almost all cellphones now have a feature on settings to not only adjust the amount of brightness of the cellphone, but also to enable "Eye Comfort Shields" or "Blue Light Reduction" settings. Through that setting you can customize how much you want to reduce blue light on your cellphone. It is also important to note that not each cellphone has the same blue light reduction effectiveness, and some cellphones cause more eye pain then others.

General Note: Cellphones are very difficult for individuals with chronic light sensitivity conditions to use. For this reason, I keep my phone off for the majority of the day so that I can limit the amount of eye pain and eye strains that may occur.

In a similar note to handheld videogames, cellphone videogames are very harmful to individuals with light sensitivity conditions. Due to the chronic light sensitivity condition which occurred in late 2020, I was forced to quit handheld gaming devices (like the PlayStation Vita and the Nintendo Switch in Handheld Mode). Because of my eye injuries, I was also forced to quit mobile cellphone gaming in order to save my eyes from experiencing significant eye pain and eye strains.

Your Custom Cellphone Settings

Use this blank space to document your customized techniques and solutions for reducing eye pain while using Cellphones (I.E How many stacked privacy screens are used & natural light settings). What are your Cellphones "eye comfort shield" or "blue light reduction" settings.

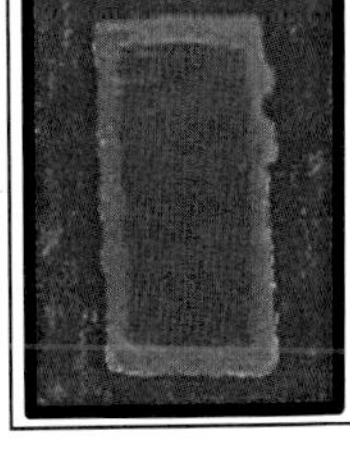

Closing Statement

With chronic light sensitivity conditions, life decisions are about compromises and priorities. The greatest trait for dealing with light sensitivity conditions is patience and a dedication to discovering techniques which reduce the amount of eye pain and eye strains that occur while doing most or some of the things that you want to do in life.

Every light sensitivity condition is somewhat unique, and that is why I created a custom techniques page at the end of each chapter for you to fill in. The settings that worked for me may be too extreme, and you may require less privacy screens and less natural light than I do. Also, the settings that worked for me to reduce eye pain and eye strain may not work for you, as your light sensitivity condition may be of a higher sensitivity.

My main attitude that I have applied since developing a chronic light sensitivity is that if there is something that is causing my eyes pain, how can I change my techniques and develop solutions to reduce the amount of eye pain and eye strains that occur while using electronic devices.

From that attitude and mindset beginning in late 2020, I learned and developed all the techniques that are featured in this book over a timespan of several years. For individuals dealing with chronic light sensitivity conditions, there is a constant battle of patience and frustration. Not being able to watch shows and movies (and also being unable to play videogames) without applying major sacrifices and adapting modified yet limiting techniques, is a very a difficult situation that requires patience amidst frustration.

Every day since late 2020, I am encouraging myself to be patient, hopeful, and to be dedicated to the process of developing techniques and solutions that will help reduce the amount of eye pain and eye strains that may occur from watching electronic devices.

Please contact your eye doctors and healthcare professionals before applying any of the techniques that are taught in this book. Please show and recommend this book to medical professionals that work in the field of eyecare, so that this book can help medical professionals better help individuals with chronic light sensitivity conditions.

Best, Russel Alden Arlotta

The End.

Thanks For Reading.

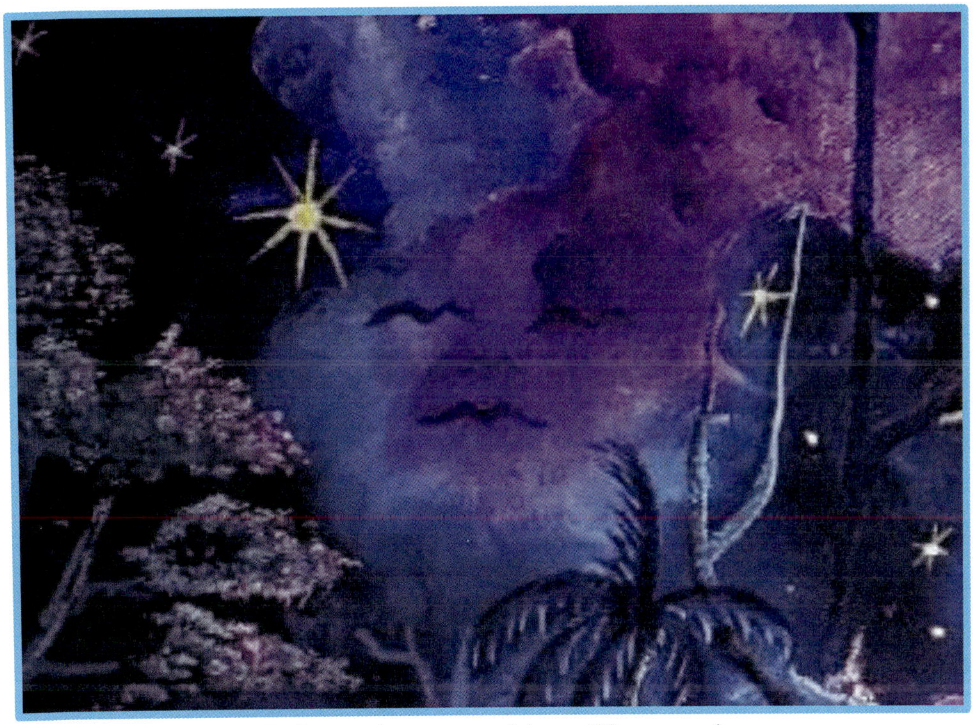

Painter: Amungwa Linus 'Kayaman'

Light Sensitivity Pain Reduction Techniques for Electronic Devices

By: Russel Alden Arlotta & Illustrated by Amungwa Linus 'Kayaman'

<u>Author Bibliography - Books By:</u>

<u>Russel Alden Arlotta & Illustrated By Amungwa Linus 'Kayaman'</u>

•*Goal Invention:*

The Mental Therapy, Sport, and Hobby

- Amazon Kindle Version (235 Pages) Available Now in Paperback.
- Available Digitally on Play Store's Book Section.

A reader interactive textbook that instructs *The Cycle Case Number Goal Invention System*, a system which promotes goal invention. Study the system chapter by chapter and perform the mental therapy, sport, and hobby of goal invention, as you become the co-author of this textbook. This reader interactive textbook, *Goal Invention: The Mental Therapy, Sport, and Hobby*, is structured in two halves.

The first half of this textbook instructs *The Cycle Case Number Goal Invention System*. The second half of the textbook contains the reader interactive Goal Invention Workbook entitled "The 10-Cycle Goal Invention Journey". The 10-Cycle Goal Invention Journey is the preformatted workbook section for you to perform goal invention as a mental therapy, sport, and hobby, while using the systematic procedures of *The Cycle Case Number Goal Invention System*.

In *Goal Invention: The Mental Therapy, Sport, and Hobby*, you perform *The Cycle Case Number Goal Invention System* and become the Author of this book.

You are *The Cycle Case Number Goal Invention System Author*.

Author Bibliography - Books By:

Russel Alden Arlotta & Illustrated By Amungwa Linus 'Kayaman'

- ***How Cellphones Cropped, Distorted, and Visually Censored Cinema: Let's Save Cinema***

- Amazon Kindle Version (164 Pages) Available Now in Paperback.
- Available Digitally on Play Store's Book Section.

Let's save cinema by applying the *Cinema 3-Step Solution*, a concise solution on how to provide consumers with the freedom, choice, and ability to consume and enjoy cinematic films across all devices and applications in their original Fullscreen contents and original Fullscreen aspect ratios of 4:3 – 16:9 / 1.85:1 without the films' contents being cropped, distorted, or visually censored.

It is time to end the forced cropping/visual censorship of cinematic films which removes nearly 50% of most films' pixels and contents on Movie Streaming Applications (Netflix, Prime Video, Hulu, & Tubi) and Online Film Channels on YouTube.

It is time to end the forced visual distortion, morphing, junking, and composting of cinematic films which reduces the size of films by nearly 50% in size (vertically) on Movie Streaming Applications (Netflix, Prime Video, Hulu, & Tubi) and Online Film Channels on YouTube.

It is time to save, restore, and protect the contents and copyrights of cinematic films across all applications and devices for the current generation and future generations to treasure & enjoy.

<u>Author Bibliography - Books By:</u>

<u>Russel Alden Arlotta</u>

• *The Detective Show Directory*

- Amazon Kindle Version (24 Pages) Available Now in Paperback.
- Available Digitally on Play Store's Book Section.

The Detective Show Directory includes an extensive list of many of the world's detective shows, consisting of over one hundred shows. In addition to the directory, there is an interactive detective show directory chart for the reader to mark the watching completion status of each show featured in the directory. The interactive chart also allows the reader to grade and comment on each show.

• *The U.K. Comedy Show Directory*

- Amazon Kindle Version (30 Pages) Available Now in Paperback.
- Available Digitally on Play Store's Book Section.

The U.K. Comedy Show Directory is a reader interactive directory consisting of over one hundred and fifty comedy shows from the United Kingdom.
With this book, readers can mark the watching completion status of each show featured in the directory.
In addition, readers can also grade and comment on the shows featured in the directory.

Made in the USA
Middletown, DE
12 December 2024

66715862R00029